MAD PR

A CELEBRATION OF MI

Edited by
Ted Curtis, Robert Dellar, Esther Leslie & Ben Watson

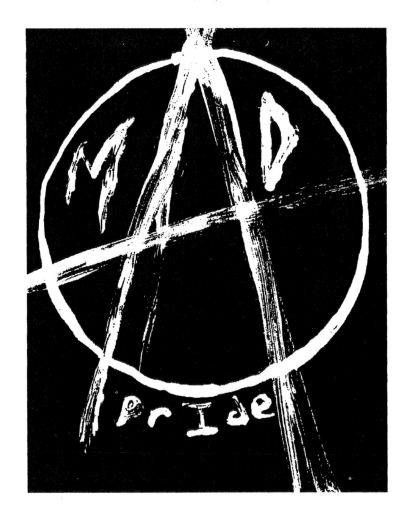

First edition, 2000
ISBN 0-9525744-2-X

This book was assisted with a grant from the Mind Millennium Awards.

MAD PRIDE
A CELEBRATION OF MAD CULTURE

Edited by
Ted Curtis, Robert Dellar, Esther Leslie & Ben Watson

Designed by **Julie Hathaway**
Cover art by **Keith Mallinson**
Animations by **Cat Monstersmith**
Mad Pride logo by **Penny Mount**

Thanks to
Simon Barnett, Stan Batcow, Ami Clarke & Tuba Karacalar

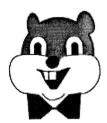

WWW.CHIPMUNKAPUBLISHING.COM

CONTENTS

INTRODUCTION

Mad Pride is set to become the first great civil liberties movement of the new millennium. Over the last century, giant strides forward were made by those asserting their rights and self-determination in the fields of race, gender and sexuality, but 'mental health' issues failed to keep pace. This is set to change.

This book is published at a time when the British government is proposing to enact one of the most despicable and shocking threats to civil liberties in living memory. The planned "mental health act from hell," as it is already widely known, promises to allow the medical profession to force-feed toxic drugs to people in the community with a mental health diagnosis, in order to increase profits for pharmaceutical multinationals. 'Mad' people will continue to be incarcerated with even fewer rights of appeal than previously, and the boundaries between 'mental illness' and 'criminality' will be further blurred. No doubt mental health system "survivors" or "users" can expect during the next decade to be charged rent by biochemical research companies for carrying patented genes. However, thousands of 'mad' people will refuse to take any of this without a fight.

If there was ever any doubt, 'reasonable' methods of influencing the way that 'mad' people are treated have been proven inadequate by the drafting of the mental health act from hell, which has ignored all expert opinion and informed debate. Engaging with government commissions and planning groups is all too often a way for survivors' views to be absorbed into bureaucratic systems, only to be rendered powerless. It is hardly surprising that a growing number of survivors operating in the "user movement" now feel that direct action is the correct way forward: defiant displays of ostentatious madness; riots; sabotage; medication strikes; and linking up with those elements who wish to bring about a complete transformation of society.

This collection documents some of these wilder fringes of the user movement. The writings which follow are written from perspectives concerned with reclaiming the experience of madness and the language surrounding it. Mad Pride itself is a group which promotes raves and rock concerts as a means of spreading the word, and while it does not wish to take part in the endless debates around terminology which have already wasted so much of the user movement's time, it asserts that language can be subverted and that words derive their meanings from the contexts in which they are used. Neither Mad Pride nor this book claim to reflect a fully-developed political philosophy, but each addresses some of the issues that will arise as we sharpen our visions.

Much of the literature around mental health has focused on the 'victim' status of mad people. This book, on the other hand, celebrates madness largely from the perspectives of users who refuse to be ground down. It asserts the rights of 'mad' people without pleading for them, in the belief that we should not push meekly for minor concessions, but instead change the world into a fit place for us to live in.

What follows, therefore, is writing boasting about the wild things the authors have done when they've been losing it; accounts of personal empowerment and liberation through madness; a few pertinent 'political' pieces; and a great number of gratuitous gestures of defiance. It suggests that 'madness' is as much to do with sex, drugs and rock 'n' roll than with the "long, echoing corridors" described repeatedly by survivor poets. And while, of course, this is far from being the whole truth, it is mindful of the tactics necessary to implant Mad Pride into public consciousness as a liberation struggle in its own right.

Some people will be offended by this book, much of which is not pretty. It transgresses simplistic imperatives of 'political correctness' which try to convince us that polite manners and portraying the world as a cleaner place than it really is do anything other than reinforce the status quo. It also reclaims the dishonest 'murderous nutter' caricatures pushed by the media and by anti-mental health groups like the Zito Trust and SANE, in order to turn popular stereotypes back against themselves. These writings mock conformity, resist 'normalisation' and refuse to be co-opted. They rejoice in madness from a standpoint of anger, humour and rebellion.

Living as we do in a world in which, as the great French poet and madman Antonin Artaud pointed out, every day one eats vagina cooked in green sauce or penis of newborn child whipped and beaten to a pulp, just as it is when plucked from the sex of its mother, madness, though usually very painful, often appears as the only available response to an obscene system. We believe that Mad Pride as a civil liberties issue needs to come to an accommodation with the wider class struggle, for each to reach meaningful fruition. We also believe that this will take place. This book is part of our attempt to make this happen sooner rather than later.

THE LAST 69 TO CHINGFORD

MARK ROBERTS

One of the things about Chingford is that the 69s don't go there. They stop well short, at Walthamstow Central station. Then they turn around and trundle back to the most forgotten and forlorn place in London – North Woolwich. All civilisation stops at Stratford, but the 69s go down through the Eastern docks and out into the wasteland. And then they come back to Walthamstow again. Day in day out, they do that.

Though of course, they ought to go to Chingford.

Chingford is a leafy suburb full of rich folk. It nestles on the edge of the people's park – Epping Forest. It was given to the people of London by Queen Victoria, with the proviso that the state could always take bits back again to build motorways whenever they wanted to.

Years ago people used to get the train out of the East End to Chingford station where they would be met by the horse brake (a horse-drawn bus), and then travel deep into the forest, where you had everything you needed. Fishing, nature trails, smooching, pony trekking – you name it. Then in the evening you could relax with a glass of stout at the Royal Forest Hotel or take in a disco at Epping Forest Country Club. No need to go to the Balearics when you've got all that.

I come from Chingford. Mum and Dad were alive then and we lived in a quiet street. Our house, which was only a council place but still pretty sought after, was right next to a quiet backwater of the forest. I would take Judy, our Airedale there twice a day or more. A bit into the forest at the top of a hill was the site of a little old house. The neighbours said that the man who lived there was a pretty strange geezer. T.E. Lawrence, he was called: Lawrence of Arabia – you remember the film. Come to think of it, some of them called me pretty strange too: but only those who didn't know me.

One morning, really early, I'd taken Judy out and the air was wonderful. It was the start of spring. The oaks were still bare, but the other trees and the bushes were so bright green it was unreal. There was a warm mist and only a few white clouds were about. It was shaping up to be one of the first hot days of the year. I had put on a fresh white shirt and a clean tie, and my uniform looked really smart. The trouble was that it was still too early. I couldn't wait to go to work.

I paced around our front room, having about six cups of tea and ten cigarettes, thinking about how lucky we were to have the forest and how few people seemed to go there. Of course they don't publicise it, and that's the trouble. You always see Margate, Windsor Safari Park and Shakespeare country advertised on the buses, but never Epping

Forest. No-one does tours to the forest. This was giving me an idea.

Normally I get on fine with the voices. Sometimes they're pretty nasty, but I never act on them unless I agree with them. This morning they were saying that I was selfish so I went and did the washing-up. Then I cleaned the kitchen, but they didn't think that was good enough. People were sad: they were waking up with the Monday morning blues and it was up to me to make them happy.

Eventually it got to about twenty past six – I was rostered for six fifty instead of the four fifty-five which I preferred. I left it as late as I could, and then I got my old racing bike out and made it down to Leyton garage with ten minutes to spare.

I clocked on and was feeling really good. My first bus – to North Woolwich - was dead, and by that I mean empty. I cleaned the steering wheel: why do the night staff always leave it covered with diesel? We have to serve the public you know, and they don't want their change all black and sticky.

Even at that time in the morning, there was loads of traffic building up and it was slow to Stratford. I could have gone down to East Ham but that was even worse, usually. I was thinking about buses – and also about how travel used to be. What about the Golden Arrow, which I went on as a kid? Non-stop from Victoria to Paris. And the Orient Express – all the way to Constantinople. It doesn't go that far nowadays, I thought.

I was five minutes late at Stratford, but after that it was plain sailing. You could get down to North Woolwich pretty quickly and I made up three minutes. The bus was a good one, the turbo was working well and it was fairly purring at about 45mph. You go through the empty docks, past a few grey estates, past Tate & Lyle where nobody works anymore, and then you get to North Woolwich. They're building a railway museum there which no-one will ever go to because hardly anyone lives in the area. But it's going to show how public transport used to be.

By the time I pulled into the station I had made my mind up. A lot of people were going to be very happy that day.

Sure enough, the ferries had just started working. Most people think that North Woolwich is south of the river in Woolwich, but it isn't. It's north, and it's connected to Woolwich proper by the Woolwich ferry and foot tunnel, where you can just about get a bike down. Lots of people come across from Woolwich and get the 69 to Stratford, and then a train to the city. Here they came now. Quite a few men in suits, women in twin-sets, a few workmen with tools – you know, spirit levels and plasterer's floats.

I opened the doors. Usually I didn't talk to people, but for some reason this morning I greeted them all.

"Good morning. Welcome to London Transport," I said. "Good morning, and how are you today?"

"Oh, he's on form this morning," said one woman to another.

"I certainly am, and that's because it's such a beautiful morning," I beamed.

And it was. You could hear the gentle lapping of the river. The birds were singing high up in the British Telecom satellite receivers. The sky was nearly completely blue. The mist was clearing and you could see the hills of Kent on the horizon.

"Not if you've got to work," said a workman.

"Not to worry. You're in for a surprise, mate" I said.

The bus was not so full that anyone had to stand – but there must have been about twenty-five people on board. I got out of the cab and announced to the lower deck passengers:

"London Transport would like to welcome you aboard this special 69, and would ask you to sit back in your seats, relax and enjoy the journey." One or two smiled, but most of them, I have to admit, looked a bit puzzled. I went upstairs and made the same announcement.

Coming down again, someone said: "Hurry up driver. Some of us have got to get to work."

"Don't worry," I replied. "We'll be there in next to no time."

We pulled away smoothly enough and negotiated the sharp corner round into Albert Road. We began to gather speed. A few people were waiting at the request stops and were holding out their arms. I pulled into the middle of the road and held up my hand as if to say, sorry, we're not stopping.

There were a few murmurs from the passengers, but I suppose they didn't mind too much, as they were in a hurry.

"OK, we're off now!" I announced, and there was no response other than a low hubbub. Obviously people were wondering what was happening. Well, they were in for a surprise. The old Perkins 12-litre engine hissed away beautifully.

"To the right, you will see where people live in absolute poverty," I told them as we passed a dismal grey 1970s high-rise. "And to the left, that's where rich people make money beyond our wildest dreams." BT's white satellite farm reached up eagerly into the skies, sucking down the latest share prices from outer space. We passed the enormous Tate and Lyle sugar cane refinery, where hardly anyone at all works any more. It's all done by machines. Past the London City Airport, which only allows little aeroplanes with propellers. Call that an airport? More like an aerodrome.

Amid scenes of desolation rather like a nuclear holocaust, a solitary plate glass building gleamed. "That's the Docklands Development

Corporation," I announced. "It plans the roads, railways, airports and anything – except what local people need. In the distance the phallic pyramid of Canary Wharf bravely heralds the new capitalism." Now, that would be a sensible place for the IRA to blow up.

The Leyland fairly glides along: not many of these buses are this good.

"How are you all doing?" I shout. I sense a muttering: but everyone is doing fine. If they weren't, they'd say so.

Suddenly, it's traffic and it's Stratford. It's slow-going for a bit. They're building a Eurotunnel-style station. Why? As if people from Milan, Zurich, Paris and Brussels all want to come to Stratford and not to central London, and people from London might get cold feet, and want off at Stratford.

Zooming up Leytonstone High Road, past bus stop after bus stop, I point straight ahead for the benefit of any waiting passengers to indicate that this is an express service.

Aha! And there is the good old inspector. 'Gadaffi', they call him. He's always trying to catch the driver out and then get them on a disciplinary. Eventually they move him elsewhere, otherwise they wouldn't have any drivers left working. He looks cross and he might turn nasty; still, he's not getting on my bus today!

Strange, I've never had a bus so full and so quiet. Obviously all of the passengers are enthralled by my mystery tour!

Walthamstow High Street – usually I would turn into the bus station here. But not today: oh, no! Instead it's straight down onto Forest Road, up to the Waterworks and then into Woodford New Road as we begin our descent into Chingford.

A strange but significant buzzing was coming from the windscreen. This meant that everything was all right – the bus was on a mission. It might even alter the course of history.

Now that I was off-route, I would have to fly on manual. The autopilot wouldn't work out here. Which way should I go? I opted for skipping Whitehall Road, which would have been a mistake, and then carried on through the forest to Rangers Road, where I took a left. No low railway bridges here.

Leafy. Green and glistening. Past ponds and streams. Let the water flow down, flying underground. Cruising easily on to Chingford Station.

"Ladies and gentlemen, we're here – welcome to Epping Forest!" I could see the passengers' eager looks in the mirror. You might ask yourself, I hummed. You might ask yourself: What is this beautiful forest? What is this beautiful station? WHAT HAVE I DONE?

A helicopter goes vd-vd-vd overhead. A couple of buses in the station: from out of town. 444s and stuff. Two London Transport cars.

Two ambulances with blue lights a-flashing. Oh, and that looks like one or two armed response vehicles, along with a police van and half a dozen panda cars. It looks as if there could have been an incident.

"We're here," I exalted. "Just go through to the forest. Queen Elizabeth's Hunting Lodge and cream teas from the Butler's Retreat up the hill."

"You've done it!" the voices hissed in congratulation.

The doors flapped open, and the passengers eagerly filed out in silence. I smiled radiantly at them, and they nodded and smiled back.

Suddenly I saw the sinister figure of Dr. Liam Duignan, consultant psychiatrist, coming towards me with a guy in a sports jacket and bow-tie, menacingly smoking a pipe. That's either MI5 or a social worker, I thought. Same difference.

Come to think of it, there were lots of professional groupings standing around nonchalantly, firing sidelong glances at my driver's cab. And at the station entrance, hundreds of commuters were not getting on their train, but were watching the professionals.

"Enjoy your day in the forest," I said cheerfully to the last of my passengers. I began to fill in the log of my final journey – the last 69 to Chingford.

Next stop – Naseberry Two ward, Claybury Asylum for a few weeks.

Well, I was medically retired, and do you know – I haven't worked for London Transport since! Dr. Duignan said I was very lucky not to have been arrested. For what? I asked. Well, there was the kidnapping of thirty-odd people. Of course that was rubbish – no-one complained to me that they didn't want to go to Chingford. LT may have been a bit sheepish about employing for so long a driver who was under a psychiatrist. Dr. Duignan could have been in trouble for not telling LT of my long psychiatric history.

And I often wonder how much London Transport had to pay out to the passengers. Not half so much as they would have if I'd taken people from Chingford to North Woolwich, I'll bet.

INTO THE DEEP END
PETE SHAUGHNESSY

I know that Mad Pride doesn't define what madness is. It's a concept which in my book is self-defining. The other day I was giving out Mad Pride literature and this eco-couple started to really probe me. Yeah, they had all the right answers, but what did they want from me? A Mad Pride badge! In the end, I said "well, Normal Steve and Normal Sue, it's nice meeting you." They both wore uncomfortable smiles. "For 750 years, people have been killing, dumping and taking the piss out of people like me. It's about time we made up on some of the piss taking."

My story is about direct action. Ironically, my road into 'madness' began with direct action. I worked on the buses at Peckham, South London for three years, and had to put up with a lot of shit there. So, when the company announced longer hours and less wages to a group of drivers at my garage, enough was enough.

SILENCE OF A SHEEP: DIRECT ACTION

I went on a hunger and speech strike at the bus stop outside the garage. Most drivers at the time said that this was when I went 'mad'. Others put it down to the iron bar assault I'd experienced earlier, going to the aid of a conductress I was working with. She was kicked in the face at 10 am because a guy wouldn't show his pass, and I got cracked with an iron bar by his mate. A nice bit of sanity! My shrink reckoned I got good value at £3,000 criminal injuries for that nice bit of sanity. My sanity for 3K. Cheers Doc.

Anyhow, back to the strike. It lasted from 4.18 am to 7.30 pm. I wrote to Simon Hughes MP, and he came to visit me. My manager came out with Hughes to try to get me on a bus. I wrote 'fuck off.' The reason I finished the strike was that I accidentally spoke to some kids. They picked up a load of newspapers that I was going to stick up my jumper that night to keep me warm, and threw them in a puddle.

One turned round and asked, "are they yours?"

"Yeah," I said.

I'd broken my vow, my personal principle. The strike was over.

Amazingly, at exactly the same time, there was a 'mad' coincidence: a memorial service started for my sister's best mate's dad, a British Rail employee who was murdered for £20 one night outside Peckham train station. That event hurt too.

Looking back at the sea of exploitation and violence at the time, it was no wonder that I took the only logical way out: to go into my 'madness'. Fantasy was the only relief. I was going through my own personal

Vietnam.

The day after the strike, I went to my GP who, incredibly for a medical person, understood my distress and gave me a six week sick note. The next direct action was to find the Holy Grail.

THE HOLY GRAIL

I picked up the 'spear of destiny' and became fixated with the Nazis' obsession with the Holy Grail and the spear that killed Jesus. Hitler's theory was that whoever controlled the spear controlled world destiny. So their cocktail of the occult, paganism and all things Jesus was Indiana Jones stuff to me. I went trawling round the Grand Masonic Lodge, Connaught Hall in Covent Garden. I then decided to find what they never could: the Holy Grail.

Via buses and train I encountered the Donga tribe, who were an eco-action group blocking the by-pass at Twyford Down. I promised a Donga woman that when I found the Holy Grail, I would bring back some holy water to 'bless' the site.

I then took to my stage-coach - the bus company - taking two days of bus hopping to arrive at Glastonbury. Walking up the road outside the town, I discovered the Chalice Well in the Chalice Gardens. I had found my Mecca, the Holy Grail. I washed myself in the well water – which pissed an old woman off as she was holding her bottle, ready to drink from it.

I filled my bottle for the Donga tribe, and went off to sample the pre-Christmas delights of Glastonbury. On the way, I bumped into some hippies who invited me into their squat. It was all idyllic: no electricity, candle lights and pot boiling over the open fire. They thought they were radical, but I was obviously pissing them off with my theories. To articulate a point I raised my arm and my jacket caught fire. Fortunately, Chalice Well water was available to douse me. The Holy Grail water saved my life!

We went into town to get some sarnies off the Sally Army and I was entertained by the hippies skanking to the Army's Christmas tunes in the High Street.

Back at the squat, two of the hippies wanted to have a shag. Two's company as it were. "Go and find Mohammed," they said.

So at 2 am on a dark December night in Glastonbury, with a massive hole in my coat, I decided to walk the seven miles back to Wells to begin my journey back to the Donga tribe. I arrived back at Twyford Down at sunset, in time to see them being evicted by the police. I poured the water onto the mud to bless it.

Then I went back to London: a new second-hand coat from Warminster and the Holy Grail having been found, it was time to move on. A Celts book in a second-hand bookshop gave me inspiration. My Celtic roots were drawing me in. I especially liked a story where a tribe of Celts sacked Rome. Their secret weapon was to put lemon juice in their long hair, which bleached it. But what really shook up the Romans was the fact that the Celts would strip off naked when they went into battle and run at them with a blood-curdling roar. This technique definitely captured my imagination, and I have to say I that I've occasionally repeated it in psychiatric institutions when the staff shout "breakfast". A nurse once dropped the cornflakes in fright. Needless to say, I got an injection for breakfast.

So it was new year. I dreamed of sending my kids into space 'Star Trek' style, but first of all there was the Irish problem to sort out. There was also the small matter of London buses to deal with. On 2nd January, 1993, I was called back to work. I was sent straight to the London Transport doctor in Marylebone, right next door to Saneline. As I waited in the reception, the date had signs for me.

It was my sister's birthday, and sadly she died nearly three years later on 2nd October 1995. Also, the 2nd of January 1990 had been my first day at London buses, and as I sat in a customer care session I had a nosebleed. I NEVER have nose bleeds – this had been an ominous sign.

Sure enough, as I sat at Marylebone, I looked back at the assault and remembered the broken nose I'd received from a wicked head-butt. I was now confined to a life of snoring and always having a bogey up my nose which I can never get out. All for 3K.

Anyhow, this doctor with a white coat called me in and sat me down.

"Listen," he said, "I haven't got you here to examine you, I just wanted to hear how your hunger strike went." I told him. He was empathetic. When I finished speaking, he said "well done, you've succeeded in your mission. You've really wasted the management's time. By the way, you're fit for work."

Back at work, they made me sit around for a day before giving me my first job on the road. At 8.20 am on the 4th of January 1993 I went to pick up a bus in Peckham. I noticed that the brake light wasn't working, so I should have called the engineer out to fix it, but instead decided to drive the bus as far away from the garage as possible. At Harrow Road Police Station, I booted the last two remaining passengers off and told the police about the defects: no brake light, no fare chart, a dummy video and, as said PC Harrow Road, a cold bus. I rang the engineer and he choked in his tea when I said "no fare chart."

"What fucking bus has got a fare chart?" he said.

"Not my problem," I replied. "In the rule book it says there must be one."

"Wait there you cunt," he said.

I had no fear – I had my bible, the rule book with me. I was now doing everything by the book!

Three hours later, a proverbial dirty old man got on the bus. I was about to shoo him away when he opened his mac and flashed his warrant at me. "Inspector Fisher, Chessington."

"What, the zoo?" I said. Fisher and I didn't like each other.

"For the last time," he asked, "are you refusing to drive this bus in service?"

Pontius Pilate Fisher then ordered me off the bus and proceeded to drive off. I reported him to the police; he was a madman.

London Transport have some weird rules. When I got back to the Garage, they told me I was self-suspended. "You've suspended me, put it in writing," I told them. But they wouldn't, and whatever bullshit they have for equal opportunities, there's a rule 22 in their inspectors' book allowing them to suspend anyone for no reason.

Eventually, my last action for London buses was to be arrested at the head office for staging a sit-in. I was charged with disrupting the Queen's peace. I never wore the uniform again.

When I got home that night after spending all day in the cell, I asked my Buddhist hippy chick neighbour if she could borrow me £1.50 for some fags. She said no – "because you've been bad." I told her to stick her karma up her fucking arse.

I had been putting lemon juice in my hair, because it was now time to get back to my Celtic Roots.

CELTIC ROOTS

I arrived at Heathrow Airport with my trench coat, paisley scarf and long hair smelling of lemon, feeling like a Celtic warrior. In fact, I was most chuffed when some guy said to his mate, "he looks like a right Paddy."

I blew my Dad's mind when I rang from the airport saying I was off to visit my uncle. "What the hell are you doing?" he asked me. When I arrived at Dublin I went through the goods to declare channel: I had a big orange with me, it was all symbolic. I had a quiet night. The next day I was to make up for it.

In my uncle's town, Naas, Co. Kildare, there is a Wolfe Tone Pub. Wolfe Tone was a Protestant who the IRA well respect. At 11 am I walked towards it with my younger cousins, and said to them "this is a BAD pub."

"That's right," they said. "When the Wolfe Tone annual commemoration is held here, it's the only pub to be shut."

"I tell you what," I said, "we'll pretend that I'm dumb."

"Good idea," said my cousin.

So in we went and I gestured that I wanted a Guinness, proceeding to drink three in twenty minutes, which alarmed my cousins, who feared I'd be paralytic by lunch – or shot. After lunch, we went to Dublin, where I must have drunk ten pints.

That night I slept in the graveyard. Some kids gave me some blankets and some Mars bars. I slept in the gravedigger's hut. Looking back, I felt rather comfortable. Life was hectic, but I felt a freedom that I'd never had before. Arguably, my last night of mental freedom ever was spent in graveyard: symbolic.

Later that Sunday night I went round my aunt's house and they weren't sure what was wrong with me. They gave me whisky which made it worse. I took to the streets again. With no money in my pockets, my journey was coming to an end. I tried to get served a free pint – no way. Some kids outside said that if I stripped naked, it would help. I took my trousers and boots off and lay in the middle of a junction. I saw a bus coming at me. I wasn't expecting to be hit, I thought he might just stop and get help. The bus swerved around me.

I got up and walked to a canal bridge. Still half-naked, I leaned over and looked to see how deep it was. Suddenly a bloke jumped on top of me, and for a split second, if you're an Oz watcher like me, you know what's going to happen next. I thought I was going to be buggered. I wasn't, but this was where my mental health file started. "Don't jump," said the bloke.

"I'm not, stop squashing me."

"Don't worry, I'll call the police."

The police came, reclaimed my trousers and put me in a cell. Well, what do you do when you're in this situation? You do what all Celtic warriors do. Strip off and scream.

After a while I was put face down on an ambulance stretcher. My ankles and hands were chained together and I was brought to my first padded cell. Welcome to mental slavery.

Held down naked in a padded cell, I still remember that female nurse coming at me with a reassuring voice and then sticking that injection in my arse.

MENTAL SLAVERY

I awoke clothed in a dormitory, similar to the open wards of Carry On Doctor. Except, of course, there was no hanky panky here. In all, I spent three weeks in ward 8A, St Brendan's Hospital. I didn't get out of the door except when I was escorted home. Not once in that time did I hear anyone laugh.

Ironically, when I woke that first morning, I heard cheering on the TV. I thought they were cheering for me; I thought I'd cracked the system. I laugh now, painfully. The system well and truly cracked me. The freedom I had found for six short weeks was now over. Everything I had felt, loved, over that time was, I was told, "all a delusion." Time to conform.

I often compare my experiences in acute care with being a cow on my uncle's farm. The cow has to know what my uncle wants, otherwise the cow gets the stick. In mental health, the stick is of course, medication. The carrot is freedom; to get your freedom you must conform, or at least pretend to conform.

Nearly three years later, I'm sitting in chair in Robert Gillespie Ward, Guys. Beside me, on my bed, sits my girlfriend and my key nurse. I cry uncontrollably for ten minutes, not bending down, not wiping tears from my eyes. I just look at the nurse. My girlfriend doesn't move. The nurse looks at me, then at my girlfriend, then back at me again until she can stand it no more and leaves. I was learning - female nurses are not allowed to touch male psychiatric patients.

I had just been admitted for punching a policeman. My sister had just been killed by her boyfriend who was psychotic and stabbed her fifteen times while my other sister tried to save her. When Brixton police let me back in the flat, they let me find the bloody duvet that she was attacked on. No warning. But where's the respect for me? I'm one of them, mentally ill.

One of the rules of my section was that I could only go out with my girlfriend. So twice a day she had to take me out, every day. At the end of the section my consultant, an Irish doctor who took the rap for Christopher Clunis, said to me "your girlfriend visits too much, it's bad for you." I had to bite my tongue – I was still on a section. He said to me "when you are in hospital, you complain a lot."

"Yeah, that's right," I said.

"Complaining is a symptom of your illness. Next time you come in, we'll ignore your complaints."

"Thanks Doc."

Next day I was off my section. As one of my fellow patients said to me on the street one day, "I had to pretend I was well to get out of there." That's the system.

RECLAIM BEDLAM

Maudsley & Bethlem Mental Health Trust saw itself as la creme de la creme of mental health. In 1997, it was more like the Manchester City of mental health. Situated in one of the poorest areas of the country, it put a lot of resources into its national projects, and neglected its local ones.

Its history went back to the first Bedlam, the first institution of mental health. If you pop down to the museum at Bethlem Hospital, you will see proudly displayed a picture of the 700th anniversary celebrations in 1947, with the Queen Mother planting a tree. Well, not exactly planting, more like putting her foot on a spade.

So, when some PR bureaucrat came up with the idea of 750th anniversary celebrations, it must have all made sense. An excuse for a year of corporate beanos. The Chief Executive could picture the MBE in the cabinet. There was only one problem: in 1947, the patients would have been well pleased with just a party; in 1997, some patients wanted more.

In the so-called 'user friendly' 90s, I thought 'commemoration' was more appropriate. So, a few of us went to battle with the Maudsley PR machine. It was commemoration versus celebration.

I think for the first time, we were taking the user movement out of the ghetto of smoky hospital rooms and into the mainstream. We spoke at Reclaim the Streets and political events. We gatecrashed conferences to push the message. I know we pissed users off with our style; personally I found some users more judgmental than the staff we talked to. They were even a few users who wanted to have their stall at the 'Funday' and cross our picket line. Frustrating. When that proposal was put to me, I lost my nut, which meant that I threatened to bring Reclaim the Streets down to smash up their stall. Because of that remark, I had two police stations hassling me up to the day of our Reclaim Bedlam picnic, and the picket at the staff ball, the appropriate opening event of the celebrations, had to be dropped.

We had our first picnic at the Imperial War Museum, one of the sites of Bedlam Hospital; Simon Hughes MP came and spoke. There were features in the Big Issue and Nursing Times, and we were afloat.

Our next event was to screw up the thanksgiving service at St Paul's Cathedral which a member of the Royal Family was attending. BBC2's 'From the Edge' got in on the act for that one, and it's widely thought that because of our antics on the steps of St Paul's - as well as stopping the traffic at 11 am with a boat forcing Tower Bridge to open - the Chief Executive didn't get his MBE. The best part of the day for me was going back with my mate Simon 'Mr Mad Pride' Barnett. We got stuck in a traffic jam at Rotherhithe Tunnel. He couldn't contain himself, so he went for a pee in the tunnel. It was such a long pee the cab driver drove off and left him!

Our next event was to join up with ECT Anonymous and the All Wales User and Survivor Group to picket the Royal College of Psychiatry. It was the first time Reclaim Bedlam had been involved in international direct action. Keeping up the pressure on the Royal College of Psychiatry we hi-jacked their anti-stigma campaign, 'In Every Family in the Land'. The soundbite I used was: "the psychiatrist is patting you on the head with one hand, and with the other hand he or she is using compulsory treatment to inject you up the bum."

We needed a target to get the anti-compulsory treatment message across. Unanimously, everyone went for Marjorie Wallace and SANE. Up until our demo, she was an advocate for it; mysteriously she has changed her tune since. 200 people turned up for the SANE demo, which shows that if people feel strongly, they will say "I'm MAD and PROUD."

People often ask: what are the alternatives to the current system and despair? To me, it's quite simple. How would you like to be treated? As an object, or with dignity? It's almost like walking up to the nurse wearing wet clothes, and the nurse treats you for a cold. The nurse then lets you walk out without changing your clothes. When you return the next day, the nurse wonders why you still have a cold.

Similarly, I'm walking around as a product of emotional and physical abuse, broken relationships, no meaningful employment, stressful housing - and I'm taking a tablet for the symptoms.

An ex-girlfriend of mine rang me up one day, and said "I want to kill myself, but I'm scared of going to hell." She had tried many times, so it was not new to hear this. I looked out of the window and said "this is hell, Louise. It can't be no worse after." She said she felt re-assured. I carried on, "when Jesus talked about being like a child to get into the kingdom of heaven, what I see it as, you are innocent, naive like a child before the child receives pain and is sprung into the adult world." I never spoke to Louise again, but she was sexually abused as a six-year-old in Barnardo's home and never recovered. I was her first boyfriend. Hand on heart, she's probably better off where she is now.

I see life as one big swimming pool. Some of us are thrust into the deep end and we manage to survive. We make our way down to the shallow end, where it's easy, boring. The people there are scared of the deep end, scared of the unknown, so they shun people like me and call me MAD. Madness is a natural reaction. The worker who abused Louise at six years old is the killer.

THE NEED FOR A MENTAL PATIENTS UNION
- SOME PROPOSALS

ERIC IRWIN, LESLEY MITCHELL, LIZ DURKIN, BRIAN DOUIEB

Originally published in 1974, this now rare document, also known as "The Fish Pamphlet," is said by some to mark the beginning of the organised 'survivor movement' in Britain as it can be recognised today, The document is therefore of great historical and political importance. According to folklore, survivor activism was at the time particularly strong in West London, where a network of squats was established to provide 'safe houses' for people in distress. The Mental Patients Union evolved during the 1970s into PROMPT (Promotion of the Rights of Mental Patients in Treatment), which eventually turned into CAPO (Campaign Against Psychiatric Oppression) in the early 1980s. CAPO went on to issue a seminal manifesto which is still regarded by many as inspirational; however, we include instead here the original MPU document, which predated and provided a template for the CAPO manifesto. Although some of the following material and the language used may appear dated, it is a timely reminder of where it is that the 'survivor movement' has come from.

"An individual having unusual difficulties in coping with his environment struggles and kicks up the dust, as it were. I have used the figure of a fish caught on a hook: his gyrations must look peculiar to other fish that don't understand the circumstances; but his splashes are not his affliction, they are his effort to get rid of his affliction and as every fisherman knows these efforts may succeed." - Karl Mennenger.

In the past few years a number of groups have sprung up in opposition to the reactionary institutions of the mental hospital and psychiatry. Ignoring patient involvement, the impetus of these groups' radical alternatives, however, have become little more than intellectual discussion points and shop-talk for students and professionals. PATIENTS, it would seem, are seen as incapable of playing any part in fighting for such alternatives.

Almost colluding with the myth that mental patients are 'inadequate', these groups have dismissed completely the fact that patients, of whom most are working class, together with hospital workers and nurses, are the only agents of revolutionary change inside the mental hospital.

The Paddington Day Hospital Protest has so far been the only example of realised patient power in this country. But this power was only directed at the single issue of keeping the hospital open and, as a result of its limited success, it collapsed without using its political potential.

WE strongly feel that PATIENT POWER could be mobilised effectively against the psychiatrist and the mental hospital, agent and agency of the ruling class, through a politically organised MENTAL PATIENTS' UNION.

WHY IS A UNION NECESSARY?

Psychiatry is one of the most subtle methods of repression in advanced capitalist society. Because of this subtlety, few recognise the dangers shrouded by the mystification of 'modern medicine'. The psychiatrist has become the High Priest of technological society, exorcising the 'devils' of social distress, by leucotomy (butchery of the brain), electric shock treatment - ECT (plugging brains into mains), and heavy use of mind-controlling drugs. The mental patient is a sacrifice we make whilst we continue to serve the Gods of the Capitalist Religion.

The heavy weapon of psychiatry, like many others, is held at the heads of the working class in order to control them. Facts show that proportionately more admissions to mental hospitals originate from areas of poverty, bad housing, high unemployment and heavy industry - IN SHORT, WORKING CLASS AREAS. The suffering inflicted on the working class through extreme material poverty, social repression, home and work frustration etc. obviously have a tendency to result in anxiety, depression and sometimes delusions as a form of escapism.

THE WORKING CLASS AND MENTAL ILLNESS

In our class society, workers are treated as mere units of production rather than as human beings with feelings. Manual workers are forced at times to react as individuals against the boredom, sterility and virtual slavery of their work function within capitalism, remaining unaware and apathetic of their role as agents of social change. Alienated from their labour, appendages of mass production machinery, or aimless producers of socially useless products, trapped in the breadwinner role between family and job, it is hardly surprising that the man who has worked on a production line for 20 years could become increasingly depressed and eventually regard himself as a 'machine' or could become so divorced from the reality of his repressed existence that he starts to live, talk and think apparent 'fantasy'. At this point he is shunted to the surgery where he can be conveniently labelled by the G.P. as 'mentally sick' and referred to the psychiatrist. But the psychiatrist ignores the social and economic cause of the 'apparent symptoms', since to recognise their importance would expose the pretensions of psychiatry which claims to locate the 'distortion' or 'irrationality', or 'sickness' within the individual. The medical profession, through psychiatry, therefore, colludes with the profits system.

In the same way, working class WOMEN are subject to this imposed insanity. Not only do some women suffer the same work conditions as male manual workers, often for lower pay, but they are expected to act as slaves to their children and husbands. The traditional women's role is that of 'homemaker', but compelled by her husband's low income, or unsupported or hounded by the S.S., she may have to go out to work. She may also be forced to work as an escape from her insulated, isolated fifteen storey council flat or the chronic conditions of rented rooms. Many women caught in this dual role feel guilty at their apparent inadequacy in the home, become depressed and unable to cope. Stigmatised by the family, school, health visitors and social workers, they soon find themselves presented to modern medicine as suitable cases for treatment!

Another road to 'mental illness' could be UNEMPLOYMENT. When workers are no longer useful to the capitalist economy (i.e. their labour value is lost), they are thrown onto the human scrap heap like useless pieces of machinery. Unemployment directly benefits capitalism, since it discourages industrial action for better working conditions and wages, KEEPING PROFITS HIGH AND BIG BUSINESS HAPPY. Meanwhile the state conveniently covers for the system by blaming unemployment on pay inflation but is left with the responsibility of keeping down the anger of Trade Unions at the increasing numbers of unemployed. So the system quickly attaches the labels of 'lazy' and 'inadequate' to some mystical proportion of the unemployed through its propaganda media - however, this method no longer suffices to dupe the more organised sections of the working class. But at the same time in increasing use, is an equally effective method which subtly stigmatises the worker (now a 'deviant' because he does not work): he is labelled 'mentally ill'. This is not difficult to do, because by this stage the unemployed worker is beginning to feel the bite, since he is not fulfilling his breadwinner role and the pressures within the family are increasing. He also feels frustration at not finding a job and humiliation and victimisation in claiming social security. However the immediacy of the family's needs makes it difficult for it to sustain the drop in living standards and they blame him for their hardship rather than the system. In this way he becomes the scapegoat for the economics of capitalism which have deliberately created the pool of unemployment in which he is trapped. Crushed beneath the mounting pressures, he becomes depressed, disillusioned and aimless. The psychiatrist does the rest!

THE THREAT OF MIDDLE CLASS DEVIANCE TO THE STATUS QUO

The middle class is not exempt from falling foul of the system. As the managers, administrators and apologists for capitalism, the middle class is obliged to defer to the ideology of its masters, the ruling class of money-barons. In order to preserve its status and security of economic privilege and the tenuous distinction between itself and the working class, the middle class must maintain reactionary values. Those members of the middle class who offend against, reject, or who are unable to cope with the values of alienated individualism (squalid private mentality), competitiveness, and 'striving for success' are seen as a threat to the class values and therefore the class position. 'Deviants' expressing their escape from or attack of the class values through 'depression', 'psychosis' or 'character disorder', having been thus labelled, add to the numbers conveniently dealt with by psychiatry.

Confronted by psychiatry the patient, from whichever class he comes, is thrown into the relationship of the worker versus the ruling class. The psychiatrists, agents of the capitalists, enemies of change, proceed to con the patient into the belief that it is he who needs changing.

Just as the poor are blamed for their poverty, the unemployed for their idleness, slum tenants for their housing conditions, and 'backward' schoolchildren for their 'backwardness', the patient is blamed for his 'illness'. IT IS TIME THE PATIENT FOUGHT BACK!

Together with other oppressed groups, patients through an organised MENTAL PATIENTS' UNION must take COLLECTIVE ACTION and realise their POWER in the CLASS STRUGGLE, alongside Trade Unions, Claimants Unions, Women's Liberation, Black Panther Groups, Prisoners' Rights etc...

WHAT CAN A UNION DO?

1. Propagandise. By leafleting mental hospitals, day centres, hostels, industrial therapy units etc.

(A) to expose:

- the myth of voluntary treatment and admission to hospital.

- the myth of treatment, and the ways in which it is used as punishment for 'deviancy'.

- the myth of community care. How social workers act as control agents, and how industrial therapy is a source of cheap labour.

- the myth of rehabilitation. How it is a process which ensures adjustment and conformity to the system.

- the myth of psychotherapy, which can act as a subtle form of control.

(B) to inform patients about their rights, minimal though they are, e.g. the right to appeal against compulsory detention.

2. Establish a charter of rights.

- the right to representation by the Mental Patients Union in court, tribunals, and wherever the Mental Health Act 1959 is implemented (e.g. statutory admissions to hospital) and wherever required by the patient (e.g. at a ward conference).

- the right to a free second opinion by a psychiatrist of the patient's or patients union representative's choice.

- the right to refuse treatment.

- the right to retain clothing in hospital.

- the right to effective appeal machinery.

- the right to secure personal possessions in hospital without interference by hospital staff.

- the right to effective inspection of hospital conditions, food, hygiene etc. independent of hospital administration.

- the right of the patient to visitors.

3. Fight and campaign for:

- the abolition of compulsory admissions to hospital e.g. sections 25, 26, 29, 30, 60, 136 of the 1959 Mental Health Act.

- the abolition of isolation treatment - seclusion in locked side rooms, padded cells etc.

- the abolition of compulsory treatment by drugs, group therapy etc.; total abolition of irreversible treatments, electric shock, brain surgery, specific drugs etc.

- the abolition of compulsory work in hospital and outside.

- the abolition of letter and phone call censorship.

- the abolition of the right of hospital authorities to withhold and control patients' 'pocket' money.

- the eventual abolition of mental hospitals and the repressive and manipulative institution of psychiatry.

4. Set up alternatives.

E.G. drop-in/ live-in centres, controlled by patients, as retreats - free from 'treatment' and 'hierarchies'.

HOW WILL THE MENTAL PATIENTS UNION BE ORGANISED?

The Union will be organised and controlled only by mental patients and ex-patients. The union membership and voting rights will be limited to patients alone. The union must be run democratically with an effective working group elected and subject to the right of recall. Outside help will be more than welcome, but will only carry associate membership with no voting rights.

Unfortunately, there are many aspects of the problem of psychiatric repression that we have not covered. Because our pamphlet is by no means totally adequate, we can only hope that one of the functions of the union will be to look closer at the situation, producing its own pamphlets etc.

Meanwhile perhaps our brief analysis will be of use in the setting up of the union.

But in any event, the time to act is NOW - there are too many fish on the hook.

A PLAY IN THE WIFE
LOUISE C.

I had some people coming to see me. They were: consultant psychiatrist - Ben Brown; social worker – Keith Caswell; and a community psychiatric nurse called Dorothy Dilemma.

My doorbell rang and, after asking for identification, I let the three people in. I was burning bergamot oil in my burner to help with any depression or anxiety that they might have been feeling.

They came in and sat down. I did not have enough corporate chairs, so unfortunately the nurse Dorothy had to sit on a hard one. "Let's introduce ourselves." We could have thrown a bean bag around and said our names, but I forgot to suggest this.

"Hi, how are you all today?" I said.

Ben: "Oh, a bit low in spirits because I ran out of vodka last night."

"And you, Dorothy?"

"Oh, OK I guess, but I am very tired."

"And Keith, how are you sir?"

"Drop the formality of sir, please Louise. You know, talking of dropping, I dropped some extremely dangerous class A's last night and I'm still seeing pyramids and goblins."

"Good acid was it, Keith?"

"Not bad – no bad come-down because I took the Sulpiride that you gave me, along with the Procyclidine."

"Yeah, it is very good for paranoia."

Ben: "How are you today, Louise, then?"

"Well, considering that I am totally insane, not bad. That is to say, I am feeling a deep sense of loss with regards to my husband leaving me three months ago. I am trying to come to terms with being a person, an individual in my own right. The pain does hurt, though…"

Dorothy: "When you say that the pain hurts, and also that you think you are totally insane, would you like to elaborate on that?"

Keith: "Yes, please do."

Ben: "Yes, please do."

"OK. My thoughts on being mad are thus: people tell me I am mad. I have been certified as mad. I take tablets for mad people. You told me that I'm mad."

Ben: "We never said that, but…"

"Hey, look, mad or not I am a person, a human being, and being dumped by my husband of ten years has broken my heart. I do crazy things, you know. I take various quantities of class B's. I keep washing my hands. I talk to animals. Some days, most days, I hear voices, saying 'Louise, you are mad!' These voices appear to be coming from a gremlin in my brain. But you told me, it's my voice, my thoughts. It's my personality, you said. Try to have a more positive sense of yourself, you told me. Have higher self-esteem, you told me. Well, I am trying."

Ben: "Can you hear any voices at the moment, Louise?"

"Yes, I can hear your voice."

"Let's take a break for a bit. You go and skin up whilst I discuss you with Dorothy and Keith."

I skinned up in the kitchen while the doctor, CPN and social worker talked.

Dorothy: "Louise! Louise, are you ready? We are!"

I went back in, armed with a one-skinner, burnt to about a quarter of the way down, and offered it around.

Ben: "Me first, I am desperate!" He inhaled deeply on the smoke. "Not bad. You haven't been top-loading again have you, Louise?"

I blushed. "Erm, it must be subconscious."

"Well, we think that you can be helped."

Keith: "Yes, we can offer you support."

Dorothy: "I will be around next Monday at 2:30 to see you, if that's all right with you. Now, stop humphreying please Ben, er, sorry, Doctor Brown."

Ben passed the smoke to Dorothy. "You are mad but also sad, a very bad girl, Louise. But maybe we're the same."

Keith: "Society is bad. It's the social environment which is to blame. And those drugs you took in the '70's."

Dorothy: "Let's get deeper, man. Wow, nice gear!"

"Well, what I would like help with, is my freedom. That stunt that you pulled on me – not you personally, mind - that stunt about sectioning scared the life out of me. It's freedom that I want. Freedom to live in a society where I'm able to be me, warts and all. I know I am not perfect, Doctor Brown. But do you lot want to tell me if you are, if you ever have been, or fear in the future that you might become MAD? I'll put the Clash on."

A STORY OF MADNESS
STEPHEN BUDD

At the end of January 1999 I moved into my new 5-bedroom house with my wife and three children. Sought-after village, good schools, couple of minutes from the edge of town, the suburbia-meets-rural ideal.

We started a new business. I was a successful property surveyor, my wife was a director of a recruitment company. Do our own thing, self-employment and self-determination. Parental ideals of family life and of course cash. The dirty dollar, the filthy lucre of the capitalist aspirational time bomb.

Two months later, Easter Sunday, I was removed from said house by six riot police, locked in a police cell, then taken to a high security mental hospital where I was behind a 25 foot fence and double-locking doors: sectioned under the mental health act for a period of 28 days.

The charge sheet at the police station had read "breach of the peace." This had required a riot van, police with shields and body armour, and a white-shirted negotiator in my kitchen, the one I had spent six months doing up while we lived with my parents. Wife and three kids sharing a house with the in-laws. Bad, but riot police in my kitchen? Run and hide, or decide that they're not going to leave without a body and give myself up peacefully? My peace of mind; pieces of my mind were no longer in place to deal with this situation.

Inside, Carlton, the mild-mannered schizophrenic, advocate of the insane, told me "don't scream and don't kick the door demanding to be let out." Five days later, they let me out. Sit-ups and press-ups in my room, tai chi, Mahatma Gandhi: he had defeated the British Empire by lying down in a loincloth, and a splash of Buddhism cured the sick man. Or so they thought.

Is he mad?

Does he need drugs?

Is he a danger to himself and others?

The three tick-boxes of the section. The mental health act. Less rights than a criminal has. You need a barrister and solicitor to represent you to get it lifted at a tribunal. My mind was now deemed to be functioning, and I left with a bunch of sleeping pills. I threw them away. I was not ill; people and things were on my case, that was all.

We ran away to the sea for a week: Devon, Cornwall and Torquay. Blew loads of cash on the get-well holiday: hotels, restaurants, the works. We deserved it; we had had a bad time.

A week later I was travelling in an ambulance to my second sectioning, deemed mad again. The goon squad had been called:

psychiatrist, doctor and social worker. Thumbs down. Out of my kitchen again. This time I couldn't escape the meds. The little blue pills and colourless liquid. They stood over me and made me take it: medication for my mind. To cool the fires of madness, and still the kindling of the spirits. To stop me being bonkers, you see.

Eleven days and one tribunal later they let me out. Not mad again.

Two weeks later, on the advice of the police, my wife takes the three kids and goes to stay at her mother's, for their own safety. I was left in the house, alone. Of sound mind, cured by modern medicine. I couldn't stop moving, awake at dawn. Driving the demons from my head. Running. Scared, in madness, but functioning. A man. You knew something was up: feared you might actually now have lost the plot like they had all been telling you that you had. Run, again? Where? Bangkok, Ireland, Exmoor? Stay at home going into this thing; go into the archetypes, all your worst fears realised? Psychotic?

My thoughts and emotions not based on reality: that's psychosis. You know the one, the mad axe-wielding murderer: that's who they say you are. Me? Just having a bad time, I can work it out, work it through, struggle through to the knowledge, the white light of understanding. You have to work to the good stuff. Madness? Leave me in the peace and quiet of my own mind.

Two weeks later I am in a police car starting my third section. This one is for six months and includes compulsory medication. They let me out twice before: I conned them, the articulate maniac talks his way out of the nut house when in fact he really has lost it this time.

I go AWOL three days later. I walked out with a bare-footed schizophrenic hippie. I was carrying a bag with six pairs of shoes, believing that the correct footwear would enable me to survive any encounter. We made it back to his place. I believed this guy to be a reincarnation of Jesus. I believed he could transport me in time and space into a wine bar where I would no longer be mad, everything back to normal. I thought that if I stepped through his patio door into the garden, I would be stepping into a crowded, people-filled bar. I then realised he had left the gas on and the whole room was filled, thought we were going to explode, left, and stopped at phone boxes waiting for the four-wheel drive vehicle which was the mystery taxi that would contain the people who would understand, and explain that it had all been a difficult initiation exercise into the secret sect of the all-knowing.

I am returned by a police car, the one called to a disturbance in the pub car park. So this time, when he says he is leaving, says he doesn't need to be here anymore and that there is a four-wheel drive taxi waiting for me, six nurses jump on me and give me the syringe in the arse. No choice left. The chemical straightjacket had been applied. I wonder how my kitchen is getting on?

At this point my ego dissolves, absolved of responsibility and liability for my mind. Freedom to fall into an empty space where this nagging concern that something was up has lost its grip. Game over.

I sat in a chair for three days staring out of the door, unmoving. On my first arrest, six riot police had encircled me with their shields; as the handcuffs had been clipped on, the same sense of loss, disempowerment, yielding to brute strength, tai chi of the meek had come over me.

My wife visited every day, the toughest of my friends risked a visit to the sanatorium, the asylum: place of safety and protection, especially to the mentally ill. The meds came four times a day. I was so mad that the other patients seemed normal, so used to existing in the altered reality I had become. All that tripping on magic mushrooms and LSD had meant something. How had I got here and how was I going to get out?

These two questions concern your immediate past and immediate future. You had entered into that sought-after meditative state, the moment of now. Living in the moment of now, in an essential survival battle. You must not give in to the overwhelming feelings of discomfort, and you must certainly keep your concerns from the nurses. Anything that might make them keep you here longer should stay out of your observation report book. Your consultant would note all poor behaviour and response to medication at the end of the week.

At the beginning, I put bits of bread in my cheeks to soak up the liquid anti-psychotic and sedative drugs they were giving me. I was still not mad, see; still going to work this thing out for myself. Beat the system.

You sign on, struggling through forms for sickness benefit in the nut house. Your new business has failed, all your savings ploughed into the house and business start-up costs. Your house is on the line, the one that cost you your sanity to acquire. You are in the system, a new system, and you are sick. Still in mania. A maniac, maniacal, manacled to the hospital, driven from bed at 5.30 am to walk the woods at top speed for two hours before breakfast. Forced again to do tai chi looking at 25-foot fences. Discovering that if you shut one eye you could see a whole daisy in the field on the other side of the wire and not see the wire. Almost see your freedom and sanity.

You stand in line for bedtime medication with the sickest of society. The ones who couldn't take the pressure and either went down into depression or up into mania. Or was it their sickness, not their minds that had gone? The sickest will be at the front of the queue for the 'trolley'. The one with all the happy pills. Three flavours: uppers, downers and sleepers. I was on the downers and sleepers; the ten o'clock treat of ending another day, you hadn't screamed that day, the white light of irretrievable madness had not engulfed you. One more day in paradise.

You are kept there for two months. He persuades them that he is a good boy now and will take my medicine and change the anti-psychotics, the ones that will stop me having disturbed thought processes, from the liquid into the tablet. Each day then I perfect the mimic swallow as the pill is hidden in my cheek waiting to be spat out. I am still not mad, you see, and will beat this thing and understand it and so all my hidden demons and myself. I will not let some drug take the credit for all this pain and hard work. I go higher. Walk the woods longer, struggle through tai chi forcibly, counting breath to bring myself down. Kill the dynamo in my arse. The sleeping pill at the end of those days brings exquisite pleasure.

Dawn and mist rising, insight, once you realise, achieve perspective, reality context into a past state of madness, you are no longer mad, just mentally ill. Insight, insight into your condition. Something Buddhist monks achieve after hours, months, years of contemplation and meditation, that protestant work ethic applied to your mental stability. You have to work at it: no pain, no gain. How could these nurses and doctors with their tick-box assessments and their selection of three suitable chemical drugs know the answer?

Their definition of insight seemed to be to give up, admit you are wrong and take the meds. Understanding of any of the underlying causes, the holistic approach to mind and body and spirit, was not on the agenda.

But then, when the mind is running on overtime with paranoia, the twisted view of the persecuted is all that flows from the gibbering lunatic: "pressured speech" in psycho-babble labelling parlance. What weight can be placed on his words? Very ill, that's what he is, very poorly, just St. Vitus fire dance of the mind. The mystic moving in the godlight of the vision. All cultures have their madness. Many times it is transfigured into the religious context. Controlled, supported, boundaries set and assistance given. Insight? The great, the good, the well-meaning and the lost souls seeking understanding of their own mental pain who make up the psychiatric profession do not instil a great faith into 'their' meaning of the word insight.

Another tribunal hearing. Three more people to persuade that I am no longer mad. That I am better, have insight into my condition and of course will take my medication. This is the seventh time in three months that I have been before a group of three individuals who have the power to withhold my freedom on the grounds of insanity. Bi-polar affective disorder, BAD for short was my label: manic-depression. Was I no longer manic? Was I safe to be allowed home to my wife and kids? To face the neighbours,

who had witnessed a trail of ambulances and police cars to my house,
and the twitter of the playground gossips about the madman at the
end of the road?

I had the same solicitor as before, who specialises in mental health and
getting people's sections lifted. I was asked the same questions about how I
felt and did I have insight, whilst being watched closely for signs of mania.
Deep breathing, open body posture: mirror the other person, all those
business skills now being put to good use. To get me out. They had let me go
twice before, I'd been such a bad boy and conned them all. I promised I
would stay for as long as my consultant quack recommended. Plea-
bargaining. Better that than have them not lift the section and then have to
wait another six weeks for the next hearing.

They let me go, said I was normal, back to how I used to be. Brilliant. I
was knackered, brain fried on powerful pharmaceuticals, body lean and
exhausted by constant movement. Not mad now. One thing I do now agree,
after, retrospective view and all, is that I was completely bonkers for a bit. I
needed the meds and the fences, now I don't. This is a much better place to
be. Emotional enema over.

HOW I BECAME A CLOSET NUTTER
TERRY CONWAY

I can't say for sure when the journey to Friern began, but two dates that spring to mind are July 5th 1957 and Friday April 13th 1972.

My memory of that day in July starts with two policemen coming into our flat and talking to my mum. Shortly afterwards she became distressed and began to cry. I ran over to comfort her and wrapped my arms around her legs, being only five at the time. Later on I learned that the policeman had told my mum that my dad had drowned having one last dive at Highgate pond. He must have hit his head on the bottom.

My brother Gerry, twelve at the time, had been with my dad. When my dad failed to resurface Gerry ran all the way home, about four miles. I shudder to think of the impact this must have had on Gerry. As for me, being only five I couldn't understand what was happening. All I can say is that to this very day I have no memories of my father's physical presence, perhaps because I chose to forget what was painful and inexplicable to a young mind.

During childhood, I suppose I could have taken a variety of different routes that would have taken me far away from Friern Barnet. But after starting work on building sites at 15, I thought 'fuck this for a game of soldiers, I can't handle this for another fifty years' and began the ever-quickening march to Friern, the beat of the powerless thought 'something's gotta happen' keeping me company. On the night of Friday the 13th of April the march became a mad dash.

This is the story of the signposts en route to what happened during and after that night.

The evening began in the Compton Arms, as it had done for the previous couple of years. The Compton was a classic Islington pub. As you approached it from Islington Park Street the first thing that struck you was 'YE OLDE ENGLISH PUB' written on the side. Except in its mock Tudor architectural style, this was where all association with tradition began and ended.

What made the Compton untraditional was the clientele. Responsibility for this rested with the landlords Fred and Bernard, a gay couple. At a time when homosexuality had only recently been legalised and many were still protected by their closets, the straight customers acted as a 'beard' of sorts, deflecting unwanted attention. But this is unfair on Fred and Bernard: perhaps they just enjoyed a mixed crowd, or any crowd for that matter.

Me and my mates had our own part of the pub, like a back room, to the rear of the kidney-shaped main bar where the other regulars hung out. The back room consisted of wooden tables, two-seater benches and half a dozen stools, all replica olde worlde. A large window occupied most of a wall; it had dimpled glass, and a large extractor fan at the top, which proved useful when dope was smoked. All of this was packed into a 12 by 12 space, creating an atmosphere of intimacy. When the place was packed it was just as well you knew everyone.

It's funny how the Compton became our regular haunt. Before that, the Tottenham Royal dance hall had seen most of our custom. Two more totally different places you couldn't imagine. The Royal was a place of high fashion. I would parade myself in my black mohair suit, with tie and matching pocket handkerchief and a pair of brogue shoes, arriving in a crombie or sheepskin overcoat in the winter. There we could all dance, or in my case tap my feet the night away to OUR music: ska, bluebeat and motown. All the good stuff you never heard on the radio, or if you did, you'd heard it six months before everybody else.

Once in a while the motown roadshow came into town. I'll never forget seeing Stevie Wonder when he was 17 - a year older than me - at the Royal. He wore a silver mohair suit. The band leader had a difficult job containing Stevie's enthusiasm. Stevie would perform his solos on all the instruments he could play, getting carried away to the extent that the bandleader had to go and tap him on the shoulder to get him to stop, and then lead him back to the mike stand to sing the rest of the song.

What made us desert the Royal in favour of the Compton was evolution, the late sixties being fast-changing times. This and the fact that my mates needed places other than the Royal to take the birds they'd pulled. As for myself, once the relationship I had from age 16 to 18 with Sal ended, speed gave way to acid on my Friday nights out with my mates Paul and Joe and a whole new world opened up, although probably I would have swapped that world for another girlfriend any day.

At first, what that world mainly consisted of was smoking dope. Prior to acid, every time I tried dope it had no effect at all, apart from the time when my mum came home early from bingo and found me and Sal trying to get high in the front room. Mum was so shocked that all she could say was "you've been smoking pop and burning jog sticks!" while we hurriedly removed the evidence.

The first time I smoked dope was in 1964. I was about twelve and had bunked into the Carlton cinema in Essex Road with Billy Butler who lived in the flat below ours. Billy was two years older than me and far more worldly-wise. His mates were passing along what I thought was a fag.

When it got to Billy he had a couple of draws and, with a sharp intake of breath, said "want some?"

"OK," I replied.

"Do yer know what this is?" he said, passing it.

Blimey, I thought, he's making a big fuss over this fag. "Course I do" I said and smoked the rest of it, with no effect.

The last time I saw Billy Butler was when me and Sam, my stepfather, went to the pub to see Arsenal play Everton and clinch the premiership in 1998. Sunday at 3.45 in the afternoon, and the Trafalgar's rocking like it's still partying from the night before; the staff are pulling down the screen, ready for the biggest match of the season. As soon as we enter the pub, before we have time to order a drink, two pints of lager appear for us on the bar as if by magic. Billy beckons us to join him on the other side of the bar, and tells me he became a grandfather three weeks earlier when his daughter had a baby.

He was obviously enjoying the novelty of his new role, and still celebrating by the look of things. But after the initial euphoria of meeting after so long wore off, Billy recalled his first visit to see his grandchild. He'd noticed that the baby was twitching and called a nurse over to enquire what was the matter.

"Didn't you know?" the nurse told him. "It's withdrawing from methadone."

Our flats in Rotherfield Street appeared to be allocated according to how wealthy you were. On the ground floor below us were the Butlers and the Wilkins, both large families with five and seven kids respectively, which seemed average at the time. Both dirt-poor, shouting, hollering and fighting all the time.

We weren't a lot different. I can still feel the vibrations from my sister Pam getting hold of Gerry in the front room and banging his head on the linoed floor. Me and my other sister Renee always ran into the toilet and locked the door until Mum had calmed things down a little.

Above us on the top floor were the Collins and Claytons, only two kids each. Mr. Collins had his own driving school around the corner, and Mr. Clayton had a job in the local brewery and had bought a car after a premium bond win. They were the only car owners on the block. The funny thing was that Mr. Clayton never drove his car, only polished it. He even put a cover over it in the winter. The top flats were in pristine condition, just like when they were first built in 1953, but by the time you got to the ground floor it was like a bomb had hit. Hardly surprising, given that the whole place was swarming and vibrant with kids, not just our flats but the whole area, much like where I live now in Hackney.

Next door to us were the Laycocks whose older kids had moved out leaving one young son left at home. When the bloke in the house next door to the flats got shot and staggered up the stairs to collapse on our landing, I told them to phone for the ambulance. They were the only people I knew who had a phone.

We lived at number three: Mum; Pam, eight years older than me and like a second mum, Gerry, 13 months younger than Pam; and Rene, 14 months younger than me, although she never acted like it.

So you can see where we stood in the social order of things, not that we were aware at the time, but I can see now why when my youngest daughter did a primary school project on the Victorian era she asked me what it was like. Most kids in my day had their arse hanging out of their trousers. Some kids wore wellington boots to school winter and summer because they had nothing else to put on their feet. A young girl in the block round the corner had rickets due to malnutrition. A visit to the de-lousing clinic still haunts me now, 40 years later. But it was all good character-building stuff.

Amidst the bomb ruin sites that were our playgrounds, an old tenement survived, Ebenezer Buildings, I kid you not, where there was a bit of local sport when the local greengrocer sent over his Jack Russell, a rat catcher. Suffice to say that the whole deal had a dickensian feel.

See, it's true, that stuff really does give you flashbacks!

So there we were, three twenty year olds going nowhere fast, about to drop another Friday night microdot - if we could find it: they really were that small. When we were skint once, we actually managed to dice one into three tiny pieces and licked the ends of our gigantic fingers, not expecting much from putting next to nothing into our mouths. With pleasant surprise and wonder we all tripped out, but instead of a full-blown twelve hours it was more like four. Just enough to make the Procol Harum all-nighter at the LSE very interesting.

I'll never forget the first time we did it together: me, Joe and Trevor, who was the young drummer with Paul's band Mad Alice. Trevor was a nice, innocent kid who didn't come out much on Friday nights due to the tight rein his girlfriend Moira held him on. That and his love affair with the drums. He once said that if he had to choose between Moira and the drums, the drums would win. Moira understood, of course. It was that sort of dedication that led Trevor eventually to become a session musician. It was inexplicable to us that he could choose the drums over Moira, because she was so attractive, particularly when she wore her red satin hot pants, which were so tight they looked like they'd been sprayed on.

I suppose Trevor was the ideal companion on our first hallucinatory trip. His hairstyle and demeanour reminded me of Harpo Marx, except that he spoke. Harpo might have sounded similar, if he'd had a cockney twang.

We scored the acid at the Old Kings Head in Blackfriars Road which had quite a reputation, all manner of drugs being hawked openly on the pavement outside, the inside being too crowded to move. Such was the rarity of a drug den at the time that it was only a few weeks later that the News of the World done a shock horror exposure story on the place.

We dropped it at eight in the Compton. By nine the place was still dead, so we went across Upper Street to number 209, the Hope and Anchor, which was still awaiting its fifteen minutes as a leading pub rock venue in the late seventies. *The Pusher* by Steppenwolf started to play on the jukebox, and simultaneously with the phased guitar opening we all started hallucinating. We looked at each other with eyes as big as saucers and exchanged smiles that betrayed sensual pleasure and terror in equal parts. It was the most powerful whooshhhhh! imaginable. The old pub, with its fisherman's nets and associated seafaring paraphernalia hanging from the ceiling, seemed like the perfect place to start our voyage into the unknown. Before this time, me and Joe must have had diluted stuff, without hallucinations, like speed only more powerful. Once we'd managed to confirm verbally our airborne status, not easy when your voice is slipping in and out of phase, we alternately ambled and floated back to the Compton where we met Paul.

Christ knows how we'd started that trip without Paul. He was at the centre of most things that went on at the Compton. At the time, he was still justifying the title we conferred on him when we left school in 1967: "man most likely to succeed." We thought Paul had what we could only dream of: artistic talent. While most of the kids in our class were learning how to draw a prick and a pair of bollocks as quickly as possible with one swift squiggle in order to defile the pages in classmates' exercise books, Paul was in a different league. Equally quickly, he could draw wickedly accurate and cruelly funny cartoon caricatures of anyone in the class. Paul also played the guitar and wrote songs; these talents were unheard of amongst his peers, making Paul unique. The only instrument any of us were able to get anything out of playing was the said object of our quick-on-the-draw skills.

Paul eventually took us back to his attic in his parents' house, where we normally ended up getting stoned and making tapes. When covered up, Paul's small electric fire made a distinctive snare drum sound enabling us non-musicians to join in. Paul had just bought the Pink Fairies album *Never Never Land*, which wasn't about hire purchase geography but was an acid rock 'n' roll classic. It revealed its full potential as the soundtrack to our experience that night. We listened to it again when we tripped the following Friday and the Friday after that etc. etc. until Friday April 13th 1972.

Once again Paul, Joe and me ended up in the attic. It was cosy, but I felt claustrophobic because it inhibited the full range of the acid experience. The icing on the cake was when Joe refused to go to the toilet on the landing below for fear of bumping into Paul's Aunt May, who had Downs Syndrome. He proceeded to piss into a pint glass and became increasingly hysterical as it approached the top, whining "what am I gonna do? What am I gonna do?" before reaching the cliff-hanger and stopping before it overflowed.

To show how pathetic I thought Joe was being, I announced that I was going to the toilet. Under the circumstances this was like the geezer from the Scott Antarctica expedition saying "I'm going out alone and I may not be back for a while," never to be seen again. No doubt after encountering Aunt May. So I went to the toilet. Now, a piss has to be special if you can recall it 27 years later with crystal clarity. Mind you, I also remember an unbelievable pony on acid, with a richard the third that felt the size and shape of a rugby ball, but I won't go into that now.

I managed to get there without encountering anyone or falling down the steep stairs. When I entered the toilet, which I'd used on numerous occasions before, I became aware of the wallpaper for the first time. Normally it was non-descript, consisting of lots of small pastel-coloured squares. The colours as you would expect were now rich, intense and vibrant, but to the extent that the wall was ALIVE and fluid, flowing to decrease or increase in size, wave after wave, with different colours and patterns emerging each time. It was difficult to concentrate on the task in hand.

Fresh and triumphant after my epic journey I proposed we go for a walk. We hadn't been outside on acid since our first fully-blown trip when we hadn't known what to expect. We either went to an all-nighter or back to Paul's. The thought of leaving the experience open to chance encounters was unheard of. There was another local crew that tripped out at London Zoo, but even they always took some mandies with them as a bit of insurance.

In awe of my feat I suppose, Paul and Joe agreed and we collected our gear and went. Our gear included some dope we'd scored earlier, although we weren't expecting to have the inclination or wherewithal to roll a joint outside. I remember walking along Holloway Road and because my laces were undone, my shoes kept slipping. The laces became chains, I thought of slaves with their feet in chains and for a while I became a slave. Not for long, but long enough to feel the horror of it, and yes, you've guessed it, the trip was starting to turn, a left turn, in fact, up Fieldway

Crescent and onto the edge of Highbury Fields. I took this as my cue to sing *Strawberry Fields Forever* at the top of my voice. I suggested that we all held hands, and Paul and Joe were too freaked out to refuse.

I was attracting attention to myself. I can imagine what was going through the minds of the law when they turned up in their patrol car. I was so far gone that I didn't see them approach. All of a sudden out of nowhere, this young copper was asking me to empty my pockets. A split second before I was asked, out of the corner of my left eye I saw Paul empty his pocket to the floor for a purpose which escaped me at the time. The copper with him just bent down and picked it up.

Meanwhile my gaze returned to study my copper. Not so much the features, which appeared to be anxious, but the head, which was mildly pulsating. In particular, the veins on the temple, and the small beads of sweat which began to appear on the brow. My close encounter with the alien species lasted a couple of seconds before we were whisked away to Blackstock Road nick.

In the blink of an eye I was on the floor of the cop shop singing a medley of Beatles numbers, all of which had profound meaning like "I wanna hold your hand" and so forth. I belted the songs out at the top of my voice, this time with the cavernous nick as an echo chamber, improving the quality of my performance to the extent that they called the police doctor to listen as well. He must have been impressed because he went down on his hands and knees to listen. Just in passing he also shined a light in my eyes to see if I'd overdosed.

After the doctor left, the desk sergeant became pissed off with the racket and shouted "if you don't stop that fucking row I'm going to kick you straight in the bollocks!" This had an immediate calming effect on me. Later on, Joe told me that he'd really enjoyed the singing, although I think his critical faculties had been somewhat impaired. Mind you, I do feel that I'd let rip with a certain amount of soul and passion; tortured soul singing.

And then they took our shoelaces - no, I didn't break into *Take These Chains* - and put us into separate cells until about 9.30 in the morning.

Well, that was about it really, apart from going mad.

Not straight away, but the blue touch-paper had been lit the night we got busted and it was just a matter of time before I took off.

Normally after tripping I'd feel sharp, as if all the cobwebs in my brain had been blown away. Then as I parachuted down gently, the feeling would slowly diminish. Not this time: the sharpness remained, and I was slowly taken over by something outside the realm of my normal experiences.

At first I felt a creative energy which resulted in the first tape I'd ever made outside Paul's attic. Joe and Clive, another dopehead from the Compton, were also involved and we did an upbeat little ditty called *Why? Why? Why?* Much to my amazement I can still remember most of the lyrics. It was about the night we got busted and my mad interpretation of the night's events. I was starting to lose my grasp of conventional reality and replace it with a different, far more interesting version.

This losing my grip stuff also included me trying to explain to Gerry what's it all about. I thought words were insufficient so I played him a particular section of the Fairies album which sounded like the soundtrack for some form of space travel.

"See, that's what it's all about!" I announced proudly. The 'it' and 'all' I kept referring to were just everything, you know, life! You could tell that I definitely had it all sussed.

Things reached a head about two weeks after the bust, when family concerns for my well-being led to my brother inviting me to his place for the weekend. Now please forgive me Gerry, but at that point in our relationship this was guaranteed to drive me mad. Probably knowing this, I accepted. We weren't close, you see. Not only was there the seven years age difference, also Gerry and his wife Brenda had spent a few years in South Africa and Bermuda, so I hardly knew them. On top of this I hadn't quite recovered from when we grew up together and Gerry used to pin my shoulders down with his knees and slap my face from side to side. My cheeks used to get so hot that you could fry an egg on them.

He lived on the tenth floor of a block of flats on the Thamesmead Estate in Woolwich where part of *Clockwork Orange* was filmed. It was an apt backdrop for the scenes of madness that were about to unfold. On the drive there Gerry gave me this motivational pep talk, but in my state of mind it just sounded like weird shit.

When we got to his place I felt most uncomfortable with the prevailing atmosphere. I mean, what do three people who don't know each other and have nothing in common sit around and do or talk about? If we'd gone to a pub this situation would have led me to drink too much in order to relax. I didn't have a drink, but as usual I had some dope.

I didn't want to smoke it in front of Gerry and Brenda, so I decided to eat it. I don't know how much hash I ate but it was a lot and I must have been desperate because I ate all of it, even though it tasted foul. This did the trick nicely, and any blockages to full-blown psychosis were quickly removed. I must already have been quite far gone when due to my bizarre behaviour - don't ask because I can't remember, maybe I was frothing at the mouth with half-digested hash - my brother called our brother-in-law Bill to come over straight away: he lived with my sister Pam in nearby Erith.

Again, forgive me Bill and Brenda, I was soon surrounded by the three people in the world who made me feel the most uncomfortable. But I don't think it really mattered who I was with for what turned out to be a nightmare trip lasting perhaps sixteen hours, though I wasn't looking at my watch. It started at Gerry and Brenda's, but for some reason I ended up at Bill and Pam's the following day. I suppose they couldn't handle me any more, and eventually they called the ambulance to take me away.

What struck me about the ambulance was that you could see through the darkened windows once inside. I could see Gerry following in his tiny silver racing car. I'm not sure if this is my personal mythology, but I think we went initially to the Hackney Hospital where I was given liquid largactyl, which always sounded to me like a dinosaur, before being sent on to Friern.

Friern was so imposing and inhospitable that it was guaranteed to make the sternest souls shit themselves. On the way to ward 15, I remember passing briefly through the lobby where there were huge oil paintings depicting tortured souls. To get to any ward you had to go via the corridor, which I'll never forget. I'm told it has a preservation order on it because it is unique. It's half a mile long with a dimpled ceiling, and you can imagine the sounds that echoed there even in the quietest moments in what was the largest psychiatric hospital in Europe at the time.

I spent ten days there before convincing them to discharge me. I was only out for a week before I went mad again. This time they weren't taking any chances and it took me ten weeks to get out, by which time I didn't want to be discharged, much to my eternal shame. I had my 21st birthday during my second stay inside; they didn't give me the key to the door.

I remember little snapshots of my time at Friern. I recall being fed by a nurse, presumably due to being catatonic at the time. It was the closest I've come to an out of body experience, although out of mind would be more accurate.

I attended out-patients appointments every two weeks for my modecate depot. A junior doctor would briefly ascertain how I was doing. Half hoping I'd be re-admitted, I told him I'd been doing some speed. He asked how much and I gave it to him straight. "Well, don't take too much" he replied, looking at the queue of people outside. This went on for nine months until I was told not to come back. That was the end of my psychiatric career.

That was really the end of it as far as my family and friends were concerned. I'd set off thinking that something had to happen, it happened and then it was promptly forgotten by those around me. I understood where they were coming from, but I was forced to bury the biggest event of my life, just because I'd rattled a few cages during the time that I'd escaped from mine.

And so it was for twenty years until April 1993, when I saw a little article in the Hackney Gazette asking for volunteers. I was unemployed at the time and looking for voluntary work, so the article caught my eye. What's more, they were looking for people who had used psychiatric services to work in Hackney Hospital. I couldn't believe it. At last I had the opportunity to reclaim my experience and put it to good use.

I've been doing that now for the last seven years, getting ever deeper into mental health work. I even make a living out of it. I'm still a closet nutter as far as my colleagues are concerned, but my experiences undoubtedly affect my perspective on mental health and the way I do my job. Yes, I'm now a psychiatrist.

A LOVEABLE CHARACTER
HUGH MULHALL

Having realised that all I needed was a pair of sunglasses to be a world famous superstar, I hurled myself through the doors of Hackney Hospital determined to reach Poundstretchers in time to purchase this most essential of all accessories.

As I stood outside the hospital in the wind and the rain, the doom and gloom of that Victorian institution looked far more ugly than any Dickens adaptation I'd seen on telly. I crossed the road to the phone box to let the Divine Ms Thing know I'd escaped (if only on a temporary basis), and arranged to meet her later that evening for 'Hamfisted' - a night at the Spreadeagle in New Cross. It had become one of the notorious of gay venues through word of mouth rather than advertising or News of the World exposes. I'd explained to the chief nurse I would be staying at my aunt's for the night, and Voila! Free tablets and freedom.

God knows I was in need of fresh wank material, if not something more substantial, and I intended to get it. That afternoon I'd worked overtime in the hospital's cottage in a sad and desperate attempt to raise funds to purchase something more to my taste in eyewear: Givenchy, St. Laurent, Gaultier; but adding my £4.50 earnings to the state's weekly benefit of £13.50 would not allow that option.

Poundstretchers was empty as usual, most of the people in the area having far too much pride or dignity to be seen anywhere near the place. With the money I'd earned earlier I knew I'd be able to choose from their more exclusive range - the £3.99 to £5.99 price bracket - and still have enough money left for a night out. A pair that brought to mind George Michael circa 1986 caught my eye, and given that they were still in fashion in some parts of London, I almost tried them on. Instead I found myself choosing between a pair of John Lennon style reflector shades with a diamante trim and a pair of lime green star-shaped plastic shades; as the latter would only have fitted a child, or an adult with a very small head, I settled upon the former option. At last, it began to appear that maybe the sun did shine out of the world's arse after all.

I'd arrived at the hospital three months earlier in the back of an ambulance. I'd slashed my wrists and it hadn't worked. I'd spent the two days previous trying to overdose on paracetamols. I had taken over 180 of them. They hadn't worked either, so I arrived at Hackney Hospital, not knowing what else to do. I woke up the morning after having done the deed with two huge blood clots, one on either wrist, preventing the flow of blood. I could see no future worth living. My dreams, such as they were, had come to nothing, and I was about to become homeless. It seemed a strangely poetic, and yet apt ending to my life as an artist, a poet, a revolutionary, a lover. Much of the trauma I felt afterwards centred around the fact that I was still here, and my sorrow that attempts to end it had proved so unsuccessful, with my heart broken into a million pieces in this intolerable world.

Back in Hackney's Narrow Way it was now gone 6 pm, and as the rain fell I began to wonder what I would do with myself for the three hours before I was due to meet the Divine Ms Thing. I decided to pay a visit to the Space Cadets. Their scruffy and unkempt flat had become a sanctuary away from the hospital over the last few weeks, and I knew I'd be welcome.

When I arrived, 24 year old Tim and 27 year old Richard were in their boxer shorts, on the bed, playing with tarot cards. Tim invited me in, told me there was plenty of beer in the fridge and a new porno in the video, and to help myself. At that moment they were very busy, but soon I would have their undivided attention. I got a can of Stella from the fridge, stretched out on the settee and turned on the video.

I've never been much of a fan of Jeff Stryker to be honest. He's always seemed too much like someone's plastic play doll to have inspired any real interest. As I made myself comfortable, my mind drifted away from the screen and to the conversation going on behind me.

- I'm thinking of standing as a Labour MP in this area. Do the cards say anything about that?
- What are you gonna say if they ask if you've ever taken drugs?
- Tell them I've never used heroin.
- Well, the Emperor card in this position here does suggest some form of earthly power which could be to do with your career. And with the Sun as an outcome your chance of success seems well augmented, but there is no sign of any sudden movement or upheaval. It may take a while.

On the TV screen in front of me, Jeff Stryker had stripped out of combat uniform and was sticking his huge cock up the arse of some dark-haired Muscle Mary. The camera focused on his face as it sweated, and grimaced, and grunted. I swallowed some more beer and lit a joint.

I'd met the Space Cadets about a month earlier, during a previous spell of leave from the hospital, at the London Apprentice. I was drunk and drugged, slouched in a corner. Tim picked me up, dusted me down and said "you've got to find yourself a reputable dealer." It sounded like the best chat up line I ever heard. Back at their flat in between lines of coke, I first had sex with Richard and then with Tim. It was a long, luscious night of reckless abandon and the best healing I'd had in a long time.

As Richard was setting off for a fortnight's holiday in Mykannos,

48

myself and Tim decided to spend some time together. Luckily they had an open relationship. it was in the warmth of the friendship that developed between myself and Tim that I unravelled a new philosophical code to serve as guidance: to enjoy life to the best of my abilities while remembering the freedoms I'd been given, and ensuring they are passed on to future generations. It is that stance that guides me now.

- The balance card in this position suggests that possibly you need to curb your more excessive impulses and find mechanisms that allow you to take more control of your life. In time you will find a flow that allows you to develop in a more organic way, that will allow you to release your inner creativity and thereby find living a more successful and rewarding experience.

Having listened to their conversation for what seemed like an hour, I began to think it possible that they were madder than me. Tim announced he was going to prepare dinner, and headed off to the kitchen. While he was there I got into bed with Richard. Though it hardly seemed like the right time of year, he had picked up a good all-over tan while in Mykannos. He offered to do me a tarot card reading.

"From what I can see here," he said, "you have a habit of falling in love with the wrong people. You're gonna have to learn to take love and pleasure where and when you can get it and dump all the other shit." The advice dispensed, he leaned over and kissed me on the cheek, then on the lips, then all along my neck. I rose up on my haunches and as he began to remove the Fred Perry I was wearing, I undid my jeans.

Over spaghetti bolognaise I swapped half a dozen Ativan tablets and a handful of procyclidine for a gram of speed and a Mitsubishi. With dinner over and a joint rolled, Richard set off for the bath. Me and Tim got into the bed. No picture that I could show you would prepare you for his rough and rugged good looks: his black hair at a number two crop, his broad chest tattooed with a Welsh dragon, his rock hard cock, like steel sheathed in lambswool, warm, throbbing, rigid.

As they say, time flies when you're having fun. As the clock approached nine I announced I was leaving. I chopped out three lines of speed, one for each of us, and finished off the beer and the joint. A thought passed through my mind as I left their flat: Why don't I kill Rick Wakeman, torture him slowly on a pay-per-view satellite TV channel, and get rich? I was sick of poverty. Surely the six month sentence a judge was likely to give me would be fair retribution, considering the publisher's six-figure advance sum my memoirs would fetch.

The journey to Whitechapel seemed endless. The weather was no better and the sky was as dark as dark in central London can be. I was glad the tube was empty. The block of flats the Divine Ms Thing lived in resembled the Russian Gulags that seemed to be on telly all the time before the walls came tumbling down. When I arrived she was reading a copy of her autobiography, *I'm Cheap, Buy Me*. The blurb on the flyleaf said it all.

- I walked through an invisible door, a force field, an actual physical entity and since that time the world I have lived has been back to front and upside down - none of the things I believed were... are real.

The third chapter, entitled *Jinx UFO Diva Quizzes Dodgy Ham Horror*, related a tale about how having been abducted by aliens, she was forced to stand and look at herself naked in a mirror for hours on end, to a soundtrack of Dolly Parton and Tammy Wynette records. "It was pure mental torture," she explains, "and as for the physicals - well of course, at first I refused." Quoted at length she states, "by the time they'd finished with the sandpaper, and the enema, the burning wax meant nothing at all."

The Divine Ms Thing, whose entire life had been styled on the warblings of Barbara Streisand, no longer felt the need to wear a wig at home. The grey balding man who sat before me had the same intensity of conversation that anyone would have after a bottle of vodka. With a hand clasped to either side of my face he pleaded, "trust no one, no one, least of all yourself."

The following chapter - *The Psycho Vespa Trannies* - dealt with the time she'd been nominated for the Turner Prize for a piece entitled "Why Not?" - an A3 photograph of Eric Cantona, in a gold frame, with the words "sit on my face" scrawled across it in black marker. I had saved a little bit of the Thai grass that Tim had given me before I left, so I rolled a joint.

The speed began to take hold, and without understanding why, I found myself talking about Leon. How I thought he was the one, even though I didn't really know who he was. How now, after all the crap, there's nothing left but some tacky Mills and Boon novel to cling onto. I told him how I'd tried to start a revolution by dropping stink bombs in McDonalds, at which he laughed, and how it had been my ambition to one day be as great an artist as himself. I explained how one night my brain had just seemed to seize up while I was playing a game of chess; as if the burdens of the past were flooding my mind until eventually there was no space left for understanding the present. "None of it means anything at the end of the day, and as time passes on, the memory just fades away," I told him.

We didn't make it to the club that night. We shared the Mitsubishi and sat watching Disneys' *A Bug's Life* on the telly instead. Before we hit the bed, the Divine Ms Thing told me that she had heard through a friend of a friend that the man I'd fallen in love with had been a copper, married with two kids. I hadn't known or understood any of that stuff at the time,

I'd assumed that a gay club was for gay people. All I knew was he was tall, dark and handsome, and that on Valentine's day it all seemed so special. I'd felt proud just being in his company. It all seems such a long time ago now, I don't really care anymore.

By the time I arrived back at the hospital, at about 6 pm the next day, my star had dimmed somewhat. The sunglasses served more to conceal the bags under my eyes than provide cheap glamour. I got a bollocking from the staff nurse as I was supposed to have been back at midday. All privileges would be suspended, and I would not be allowed out again until they had decided I'd been a good boy. As I sat alone at the table and prepared to eat the half-cooked sausages, washed-out cabbage and other assorted stodge, I recalled the last bit of advice the Divine Ms Thing had given me before we fell asleep: "If clothes maketh the man, then the man is empty."

Suddenly I realised the whole thing had just been some bad farce. The tasteless pink blancmange that sat before me was no longer just a tasteless pink blancmange, but a symptom of the malaise - how do you make tasteless pink blancmange? How do you make anything that comes out so totally devoid of taste or flavour - or it THAT colour?

Having finished the first serving, I went up to get seconds. Is that therapy? Am I getting better?

FAMILY FRIENDS
FATMA DURMUSH

I was trying to study, but there were so many distractions, like the television blasting. A pile of history books glared in my direction. I was fifteen years old. If only I could have been reading faster from day one, but no, I had allowed it to slide; I had gone from being a good student to an unclassified one.

Then he walked in: he was fifty years old, cocky as hell and wanted to destroy me, though I did not realise it as I sat in my chair fidgeting. I had no choice but to hear him: he was a guest in our house.

He smelt of dirt and sweat, lived alone, and did not believe in anything anymore. My mother wanted to carry on watching television but she couldn't. Father liked him: we were stuck with him. Father allowed him to talk; he didn't like my mother and I chatting, for we couldn't articulate properly, but this man had my father enthralled. Mr. Salim talked on and on, for he knew how to.

He stayed until bed time. I tried to work on my essay, but he kept making remarks about it and wouldn't take the hint that he should go. Finally, I went into my mother's bedroom. I heard Mr. Salim laugh and stuck my fingers into my ears, trying to concentrate. Then he came into the bedroom and started talking. "I'm a reasonable man, but I'll stand no nonsense," he announced.

He took my hand and tried to kiss me, then he left the room. I felt the tension, but I couldn't understand. If I had been older and he younger, maybe; but he was old: what did old people want? My heart was disturbed, but mother and father wanted to sleep.

Hurriedly I thought and scribbled; I had never been so furious or so fast. The next day I presented my essay; the teacher read it and began to laugh. His smirk went right through me; he gave me 34 points.

"I'm being generous" he said. "Study writers of history, and I mean study!"

"But that is all I know!"

"Read books, and plan your essays. I'll give you another assignment later."

I was running after a train but I couldn't catch up with it, so I slept in the library after getting the books. I had to work in the cafe when I got home; how was I ever going to catch up? It was only years later that I realised how much I hated working in the cafe.

In my sleep, I dreamt of Mr. Salim saying over and over again: "Lazy sod, a lazy, good for nothing girl." And then he smacked his lips together and his gold tooth fell out.

When I went home that evening, I tried to explain to my father what was happening, but he wouldn't listen. He went about with his hands behind his back, counted the change in the till and ordered us about. Then the voices began: not just anyone's, but Mr. Salim's. It tortured me; I tried to ignore it but I could not concentrate.

I became disorientated and slept a lot. Then one day I got up, quite determined to fulfil my obligations. I began to read, but the voice did not want me to. It tried to close my eyes, but I fought. I began to have terrible headaches.

Every day I tried to write my essays but the voice made comments, trying to stop me. My handwriting became bad and I grew unbalanced. Then one day my father took off all his clothes and paraded himself in the cafe. I tried to forget my concerns and help him.

Whatever it was, was evil. I could not see the end, and it was eating up my family. Then I read a scientific book about telepathy, and decided that in order to survive, I would have to close my mind to impressions, against all outside influences; I had to fight this grave situation.

Days passed. I did not want to alarm the voice in case it grew stronger than me. I didn't go to school and I failed all my exams, but this was one exam I had to pass. Mr. Salim came and I tried to be pleasant, but the voice in my head disgusted me. It grew worse daily; I tried to switch off its power. I fainted.

When I came to, the voice was laughing and I felt like a fool. I decided to write about how I felt: I wanted to achieve something, but the voice jeered. Mr. Salim recited remarks that I had written, saying that they had been written before by other people. He also came and kissed me.

"You can't escape," Mr. Salim said. And then his bald head came closer and his smell oppressed me. I smiled at him and sat still as he felt my breasts. Gathering my strength, I pushed my hands onto the keyboard and typed. He was getting aroused, but I kept my head and typed on. I could feel the tension in his body.

A little later, mum shouted that the potato stew was ready. He left me, and the voice took over again. A headache like nothing I'd ever known before attacked me. My typing accelerated; I couldn't read the words but still I continued: the words were coming faster and faster and I couldn't get them down quickly enough. I was a box of matches, and somebody had struck one of the matches and put it back into the box alight.

I ate then I fainted. I had to carry on typing. My insides felt numb and sore. I went to bed at eleven, tired, as if I had a weight on my shoulders. I awoke at eleven the next day. I tried to read but I couldn't. A terror went through me: what if I could never read again? Or write, or communicate at all?

I glimpsed a little world of dreams before the voice jerked me back to reality. I didn't want the voice, but it only allowed me to work if I said nice things about Mr. Salim. In fact, he made my blood boil, but not in that way.

One night I was having a bath, and then I threw myself out of it in the nick of time before I fainted. That same night I woke up with my hands around my neck, choking myself. My voice had somehow discovered my dislike of Mr. Salim. I awoke bruised, but alive.

I went crazy. I underwent a complete change of personality. I had to break the chains that bound me to the voice: freedom had to be out there somewhere. It became an obsession: I sought this freedom all day, and this was all that kept me sane. I went through life like a rocket. Blindly I was reading, without digesting anything, and the voice was blocking the pleasure I had felt before. I was writing, but not learning. I was like a hungry animal denied food. My mother and I had constant arguments, although my father was getting better. Mother did not understand what was happening. If I fainted, then it was because I had to.

I was losing my grip on life: and then a sudden strength came. Mr. Salim had arrived and he was fiddling with my tits when I tried to kill him. It seemed like a wise move. He laughed at me and kissed me, and I was petrified that I might stick the knife in. And then he let go and ran out of the kitchen. I shivered, straightened myself and ran upstairs. I had to leave home, to escape. The voice in my head was very calm and I watched television. Mr. Salim left the house but his presence stayed like a sexual innuendo.

I climbed into bed but awoke at 2 am and got packed, ready. I breathed heavily and the voice began to laugh. It was going to be more difficult than I thought.

The street glared at me, and I was petrified. I had enough money for two nights. I took a taxi to a hotel, and the voice became active in the hotel room. I tried to blank out. It was so quiet in the room, and yet we were struggling. Though I did not feel anything except pinching, the voice was raping me. Then finally I cried out loud: "Get away! Go away!"

I blanked out. When I woke up in the morning the voice had left. I was ashamed, as if I'd been raped. I couldn't go back home to my father, because he would kill me: a raped woman is a lost woman. My mother would just be upset. I had to go to a hostel. The voice had gone and was replaced by deep shame; I walked with my head bowed and there was no pity in this world. I had tried to be good and failed.

Mr. Salim had to be found and made to marry me, but he had

disappeared. I was scared of being on my own. I did not want to be on my own.

Six months later, I went to the toilet and another voice spoke to me, this time young and attractive. I took my bag and went home, laughing hysterically.

Now forty, I take injections and medicines and keep reasonably sane, although because of the injections there are marks on my bottom. Sometimes I see my Kamourane, the lover of my dreams, and we sit and have long chats.

Not being attractive enough to have a proper boyfriend, I muse upon my phantom lover. The plus point in this relationship is that he is as petrified of me as I am of him. In Turkey, it is said that people like me are haunted. I am haunted by Kamourane.

Loneliness and isolation are disadvantages, but out of these my poetry and short stories grow. Kamourane the phantom is six feet tall, he has a tremendous background, he is kind and tactful and all the time he is there. Compared to him, my first boyfriend was a wimp.

The haunting began nearly twenty years ago and I've tried to get rid of it desperately. Kamourane, you are an illusion. How many times have I told you to go away?

But Kamourane never listens; even if he does listen, he makes no acknowledgements. "Eat, it's good for you" he says. When I'm on a diet, he goes into decline. "I like you fat," he tells me.

For Kamourane is afraid of losing me. He is so kind, not mentioning that my looks are average and my disposition lame, not mentioning that I have nothing but the clothes I stand in, while he is extremely talented and wealthy.

Kamourane loves blondes. Not being a spinster for nothing I have curtailed his enjoyment of blondes. We suffer each other in silence and he does not like to see me talk to men, any men, and I respect his jealousy.

At first it was as if I was dreaming. I was so happy to have Kamourane: I thought it was telepathy and that he would come and marry me. But that was years ago, and now the doctors assure me that he is only a fancy. And what is a fancy but an extension of one's mind? My over-heated mind has produced Kamourane, but the romance does not stop there. He does all the heavy work. He is good at gardening and taking care of myself and my mother. We share the typing, but he can't write, so he is my willing slave and I am the master, uneasily, for one day the slave might rebel.

56 Dear Kamourane: I see him in his various disguises, I feel his massive weight on my shoulder as I write this and he knows that I am upset. Our relationship is almost perfect, but I cannot tell my mother about it for she would be unhappy. In fact, she'd be devastated. Her little girl insane, and insanity is like a muddle, so we muddle through.

At first I thought Kamourane was real, but now I glare out of the window in despair, dismayed that there is no such person. Schizophrenia can be fun for a day, and over years it can devastate yet uplift you, and there is a pride in my soul that can never again be rebuked.

So I must say "good day" to my dear Kamourane, and maybe some day there is a cure, but not for now, and I stare outside into the birdsong of late summer and wonder: why me? There is no answer. The birds have flown, the man inside my head is typing this, and he does an efficient job as we sit it out in our mutual nakedness.

The doctor sits in the sun and I'm amazed that he can show his face and not feel naked. He drinks his coffee. If it had arsenic in it, they'd probably blame it on me. He seems well-balanced but slightly worried that I might not be concentrating. I am unbalanced, and we stare at each other. It is the way of the world that some are sane and others are insane.

"How have your been?"

"Reasonably well."

"Good. How's your writing?"

"I've had twenty things published in the Turkish papers."

"Good."

How I wish he wouldn't say "good" all the time. Maybe he has no other vocabulary? In my mind, I pace the floor. I float up and down and scream in the attic of my mind to be released: from what, I cannot say. I try to concentrate on the doctor's shirt. It is white, he is wearing a suit, and he has his sandwiches there all ready for lunch time. He looks at his sandwiches, and I smile. I am now a writer, but I'd give everything to have my doctor's sandwiches.

Sometimes I want to crush Kamourane's spirit, because he, after all, is me, and I of course am he, and there isn't even a word of marriage between us, for who can marry oneself? I fling myself from side to side, I get injected and I have my pills, and suddenly it doesn't seem so bad.

But the Cypriot community doesn't understand that madness is not always obvious, and can be insidious and deeply penetrating. So they ask me, every year when I go to see them as a form of punishment, why don't I marry?

I refuse to answer because I'm proud, and being proud, Kamourane and I have a slanging match. Oh, the things that this room has witnessed when we battle it out and the walls vibrate with anger so deep that I could suffocate under the extreme torture. And then the nurse comes and asks me what books I've read this week. And suddenly I'm motivated to read books. Kamourane can go and shit himself; suddenly I don't care.

It hasn't always been so, but now I find a kind of peace as I feel the agony of the seasons on my back and my arthritis gets worse. I realise, slowly but surely, that I'm finding my voice as a writer, and I write endless warning letters in my mind to Kamourane. He reads them with interest, the poor sod. He never complains now and we're firm friends, but years ago he used to call me a slag and all manner of names.

Poor Kamourane has suffered too I reckon. As I said, he does all the rough work around the house. Sometimes he does the cooking. He loves to cook, and also to clean his room, because he thinks he is rich and so has a sensitivity to dust and things like that.

Year after year, we do the same things together and we develop. He has developed into a nurse now. He gets extremely jealous of the other nurses' hold on my sanity and he does not like to be a powerless man, so he has grown deeply caring. Instead of the harangues of former days, now he wants to cure me.

Life is still flowing through my veins, though where to, I can't say. I gather tempo and I carry on writing. I've just written a story about asses, and the asses are the doctors who can't cure me. I get money because they can't cure me. If the doctors could cure me, I'd have to find a job, work nine to five and suffer. I write about the mysteries as I see them, and about how Kamourane has saved my life more than once. We have grown alike and precise, like two peas in a pod. Yes, Kamourane?

LAID UP.
DEBBIE MCNAMARA

This structure will make plywood of us all. And anything in-between at the threshold must go one way or the other. Did you ever go surfing? There's no need now. Did you enjoy cooking? Smoke enough and you'll eradicate those craving little taste buds. But the world turns on and there's no need to feel downhearted! If you have the stamina, you can collect bottle tops and get your prescription pain-relief for free! The news tells us snatches of the whole picture at high speed and the days have become too short to read a paper. Fact blends with fiction and we live in our own dream where there is only fantasy and no time zones unless, unless, you can carve your step and sift away, minimise your input in order to retain your sharpness, and relinquish the shadows. Can you pull away? Can you rouse yourself to reach the point where the air is clean? Do you still dare to hope that it will make a difference? Is there anything left to heal?

Remember the con of the salty soup. Maus. Fear. Ever feared for your life? Well, they've never. And now we are too tired to teach, and our brains are no longer retentive, and romanticism is redundant. Dark valley and natching of shrivelled gums! A beautiful model debauched into sallow candlegrease and love annihilation. But you know what? The flowers grow on. If you can bear to look at them, the flowers will remind you of everything. Don't get too comfortable in this maze of confusion. There is elsewhere.

One day, arriving to look upon the suffering of the poor little things as their predecessors gloated over photographs of perplexity (and maybe pick up one or two last moves) a one of the race apart sees with sudden atavistic fury that there are footprints. As it was predicted, Lilith picked up her hoard of gold teeth - her own - and walked. Realising suddenly that she'd been had, and that the only barrier between herself and life was the refusal to believe, she denounced the whole shebang as mass psychosis and hobbled off to buy a mini Sarong, and join the party elsewhere. This was no fun! Welcome to the green room. No belief, no fear.

And so the story goes: smearing butter on the dead, the gentle handled fish-knife and slow motion. In an effort to resurrect her passionate godlike man with all the enticements to recall a spirit back into a vacated body, she tempts with shot-through Marzipan, Bismark and Myrrh, greasing onto a clean pine top. She cares not if he lives, not as we know it, just so long as he is possessed of life. She is calm now after the shock and aftermath. She smears his hair with a little fat and places gold around his neck, saffron sun on his forehead in unutterable feeling, an ecstasy. She sings to the Lord in catholic prayer, the only ones that she knows, as she lauds the bones of his making and laments the freezing of his beauty.

Her weaving lasts for six days. On the seventh day she rests. She has worked assiduously on his behalf, her brief quavering, washing his succulent form in exposition of her Cancerian grief, inhaling the dust of many exhalations. She guards the lap, rests next door. On the seventh day she retires. The orchids are heavy and blue in their profusion. She has called Lakshmi, Krisna, Shiva, all the sisters in the Bible and miracle-givers of sacred texts, in writing and zither song.

On the seventh day she carries her empty heart out into the crocus morning of rude spring early growth and sits silent amid the raucous chorus, grey-eyed, head covered. She carries her material wealth around her ankles and is tempted just to walk. The wind is steady and seasonal and carries the cherubim in the sky low. Scudding eastwards. Toward the eventual cliffs. A long moment of weather changes, sunlight shafts into the late afternoon and the day is bearable. Ravens land on the silver Birch, scratch their talons and utter their guttural obscenities. At blue twilight a beam of light touches on her shoulder and her soul trembles at its junction with her being. As she turns her head he sits down beside her, glistening, wrapped in the jade cloth that she placed by him. Green-eyed he looks out at the sea of the land. Aghast with sensation, she remains simply in the moment. Her lament. The Gingerbread man. Jasmine and Nzir. There's something strange about the neighbours. Her lament has taken her heart, her joy, the freshness of her breathing. He turns to her in her pallor and smiles the irresistible smile of those who no longer ache. Something in her turns over. They kiss. He slips the tongue in. She remembers the laughter, in her own happy voice of the distance between now and the hereafter. She remembers that she ought to eat as befits the clock and she looks at him doubtfully. He offers her a slice of Bismark. She could have died laughing. All that work, and he moving. Like a magician he produces sweet almonds still in their rusting leaves, nectarines. Their lovemaking caused nutmeg pastries to appear, fully frosted, and champagne grapes to ripen.

In reeking stink of psychic trashcan wherein all efforts to maintain a sweet, sheened loveliness are thwarted, my personal battle against it all begins here, in a festering adrenal gland which, despite the ablutions involving olive soap at regular intervals, still runs into overdrive and takes my once-fresh corpse sagging along with it. I can no longer enter the kingdom of the Body Shop without dutifully masking-up at the door. Every month I am psychologically ground into some jerk's marble ashtray and I walk away from the encounter each time, determined to breathe calmly.

Valium enabled public transport to become a possibility again: but woe be to the self-medicator who does not inhabit a pharmacy. I have colluded with Diamond White and the offerings of the Jutland peninsula in order to approximate the optimum satiation of my main tantalisation and healing force, which is currently in the hands of an ex-squaddie on a mission to lose all of his friends and generally piss off everybody that he meets.

So, another day off sick, laid-up, wondering how I'm going to get my hands on my medical needs without becoming a sylvan shadow in the meantime, with heavier tread than should be the case owing to the backlog of contretemps and general hecticness in the heavens at the present time.

I have the answer. A six a.m. start and farewell to ginswilling malcontent associates seeking to be heard. A new start. A simple diet, except for when entertaining when exquisite preparation and many courses of tit-bits shall tease the taste buds from forbearance into sustained and understated climax of sensation. The year of silence and the hands. My vows shall be to be talked out, evading questions, focus outward, to concentrate fully on others, keep lists, remain with my heart, keep a cool head and a fast spark, speak my mind. And the best laid plans shall at last be realised. I look forward to seeing the flowers. By that time I should be able to smell.

There was a rock on the edge of the shoreline, chains and manacles upon it, where the remains of a servitude long past could be discovered.

I am introduced to a being I don't necessarily want to know, who hits on me hard in the "I need you" vein, and so I try and the fact ensues that I guess that I end up as being something for him, albeit not too willingly on my part. It was a wrong connection from the start. Portents warned; quadrants of the city were sealed off in the convulsions of a bus crash on their first meeting, on the second he saw somebody knocked off their trike and get injured, by the time that he had held her for a brief moment with a reflection of her own spirit, borrowed for the occasion, the Ulster Prods were emboldened enough to savage a lady barrister tooth from bone to show their noblesse after talk had been stable at tables, then presenting Engloid accents with justifications that invited the derision of the Ombudsmen and soon after India launched its first cruise after over a year of abstinence.

I approach my Sugar Loaf Mountain resplendent in the carbon-dated knowledge of this species, this supposition of every fact, life, experience and invention, its knowledge of the winds and the power of the earth, its feeling of flabby root encroachment, the thrill of buds and harvest of pollen.

Gifted are we on earth.

Today my mind is on the things of the sea, the trinkets of the ocean, the endless wheel of rotational mathematics, the waves and pools having spent the morning in quadri-dance (peculiar muscle pain for two weeks now) and feeling the need for a top-floor flat to prevent the upward-vortex suck of energy, attributable to many current factors, not least self-annoyance today at missing three appointments knowingly, laid-up again with no way to reach my medicine.

Yeah, language got mashed too - that was a while back now, and I am recovering but still keeping close to the wave. And there is just a gradual reintroduction to those echelons, and my remembrance of fantastical longings encased as an alabaster egg inside a gilded spool, within each and every atom in this, my hologram. So, hanging there in virtual space almost half-amused, clock-watching until the millennium plus fifty, sans appetite or desire or anything like that, evoking the response of a surging mass of wailing and gnashing, and the rending of nature and the squalling of lightning: like the script to the apocalypse in visual form, written up there in big typeface for the future, to play us out in style to the closing chord of the big cathode tube in the sky. And the silence before the final anthem, the catching of your last breath which we all share, all lungs united in a final gasp of exultant jubilation.

I go into my millennium with my bone structure intact, and grateful for such assets as my vertebrae. Thank you to the crawly floppy things who pushed us up and out of the soup.

ADVICE: AN A TO Z
HANNE OLSEN

(A) Never look a professional in the eye. Keep your eyes downcast or shifty, as this puts the professional at ease.

(B) Never let a professional see you in a confident state. However, if you can't help yourself, make sure to overdo it so as to fit into one of the following categories: elation, mania or megalomania. These labels are handy when professionals are asked by benefits people what your problem is.

(C) Do not shake hands with professionals. If you must offer your palm, make sure to wet it with water or spit just before, and make sure the wrist is adequately limp.

(D) Do not be passionate about anything, unless it comes under one of the categories mentioned in (B). The only safe subject is your condition and its debilitating effects.

(E) Do let the professional know that you are sometimes, when your condition permits, involved in events for and by other mad people. Such efforts professionals find rather endearing and they will express their thoughts and feelings in the most patronising language available to them.

(F) Also do let professionals know that you are socially engaged, when your condition permits, with other mad people. Not only does this confirm your malfunctioning, it cements it.

(G) If you mix with the unlabelled mad, keep it quiet, it may backfire; you may be told to pull your socks up and get on with it.

(H) For at least three days prior to any interviews involving state hand-outs, make sure you don't wash, brush your teeth, or attempt to maintain any other personal hygiene.

(I) Make-up should only be used if you are a woman or a gender-confused male, and only applied badly and caked.

(J) It is also important to think of medication. Prior to benefits interviews, do take as many tranquillising tablets as is safe. This ensures a sufficiently vacant expression on your face and helps prove your deserving status.

(K) Be very aware that your IQ is a minefield when seeing professionals.

(L) With most professionals, it is highly advisable not to challenge their assumption that you are thick. These professionals are easily detected: they will finish your sentences for you with words you had no intention of using. Their tone of voice resembles that of a parent speaking to a toddler. They laugh at their own wit. With this type of professional, say nothing, or simply agree and look thankful.

(M) With other professionals, it is almost impossible not to reveal yourself with all your faculties. These tend to ask trick questions out of the blue, in order to engage in a game. These professionals are often bored or disillusioned. With them, you are best off spending your twenty minutes playing mental ping pong, slicing and undercutting and spinning your replies to your heart's content. What you must not do is respond in a directly rational, angry, assertive or vulnerable way.

(N) If you do cry in front of professionals, let your tears be angry. They will still be viewed as signs of torment and depression, thus improving your chances of getting the help you need.

(O) Don't be frightened of your own manipulative power. It is the best tool available and easily fools professionals.

(P) Ignore the occasional appointment without cancelling. Keeping your appointments tends to prove that you are merely pretending when you refer to your difficulties.

(Q) By ignoring appointments, you get the added bonus of renewed attention. More often than not, they check you out to cover their own backs, but at least it works in your favour.

(R) There is nothing wrong with going into hospital now and again, as long as you stay clear of sections. Threatening to self-harm can be a ticket to respite in a quiet and not too harmful environment. If you are lucky enough to live in an area with supportive and non-psychiatric respite, use it whenever you need it.

(S) If your stay becomes involuntary, check out the dos and don'ts with other patients. Your aim is to stay safe while kicking up enough of a fuss to get the help you need. You are not there to be punished, although it will often feel like that.

(T) Don't try too hard to manage your finances. At least not until you have been assured reliable and long term financial help. (Should you get well enough to work again or lucky enough to find an employer, the money will serve as a safety net in case you relapse. Being given the money may even foster in you an urge to declare your good mental health to the authorities.) By trying to manage a budget that doesn't make sense, you are digging yourself an early grave. Cash in hand is unfortunately your only option to survive while you wait for the forms to be processed.

(U) Lack or loss of money, as we all know, are the triggers for depression. Get yourself a mental health advocate to help you get those benefits forms off and the appeals lodged.

(V) When doing the benefits forms, never, ever fill them in yourself or use your own words. Remember that the people who make decisions think you are thick. Indicating otherwise is shooting yourself in the foot.

(X) Beware of benefits advisors attached to social services. They are also professionals, seeing themselves fit to judge whether you deserve something or not.

(Y) Don't use words like empowerment, user involvement or self-determination. The professionals simply do not understand what you are on about.

(Z) There are exceptions, and when you find them, do treat them well and ignore all of the above. There are so few of them that, although their number is slowly growing, they tend to be over-worked and thus at risk of burn out. For our own sakes and theirs we must treat them with respect and make sure they know how much we appreciate them. Without having met some of these rare, competent, humane and intelligent people, these pieces of advice would not have been written.

MAD PRIDE AND PREJUDICE
ESTHER LESLIE

THE SPLITTING OF MADNESS

People talk about madness as if it is a known quantity, fixed for all time. But this is not so. The shape of madness changes over time, and the way it is understood and 'treated' shifts.

One time of changing understanding in Europe happened as old feudal structures jolted into new capitalist ones. In Europe, two hundred and fifty years ago, as a rising bourgeois class struggled to establish new economic and political forms, madness was re-conceived in terms of the newly important idea of 'reason'. To be mad was to suffer from a loss of reason. Curing meant the re-introduction of this missing reason, and doctors and philosophers started to believe that it might be re-introduced through useful occupation and the internalisation of order.

This marked a break with what had gone before in still feudal times. The mad had been given a place in feudal society, sheltered by and incorporated into the family, the village, or the community. New economic arrangements through the 17th and 18th centuries shifted them into workhouses, prisons and poorhouses. They formed part of a growing class of dispossessed, and they were not sufficiently distinguished from other categories of rulebreakers – the poor, beggars, criminals – to warrant special institutions. But by the end of the 18th century, attempts at reform were undertaken. The mad were removed from everyday life. They were split off from other deviants and placed in special homes, where it was hoped that healing might somehow take place and reintegration into society one day occur. Doctors were introduced to mad houses. These places were often built far away from town centres so as to afford greater isolation and a concealment of those called insane. Where in the late Middle Ages, madness was an experience capable of expressing essential truths about the world, in the period of the Enlightenment, it was more often silenced and hidden, for there could be no truth in those realms where reason did not rule. Only what was reasonable could be true.

REASON AND THE SORROWS OF THE YOUNG BOURGEOIS

Before 1600, official discussion of melancholia and mania remained fixed within the perception of the four humours and the qualities that dominate when the humours are not in balance. But after this time, the focus was no longer on the body with its production of bile and juices sending people out of control. Rather, it was the soul that was to be scrutinised. No longer was it a question of the physical substance of the humours and their effects on action, but a question of ideas and the mind. Physiology was swapped for pathology. The myth of the humours disappeared, and psychological interpretations took their place. For example, that which had previously been interpreted as hot and cold tensions in the body changed into the idea of an exaggerated accuracy of internal impressions, an overly rapid association of ideas coupled with distraction from the external world. Most important in this new idea of madness was the concept of reason – for the Enlightenment's pivotal idea was that each man possesses reason, or else he is not fully a man.

There were few medical-scientific theories of mental distress. The dominant idea was that 'the passions' were the cause of all disturbances. Madness was brought on by an excess of passion, a passion that was unbridled by reason and probably triggered by unhappy love. Madness and melancholia fascinated the German literati in the 18th century. Hospital, prison and mental asylum visits belonged to the itinerary of most educated people staying in a strange town.

A literature on madness began to be produced, and it reflected the governing ideas of the time. Suicide was judged mostly to be a consequence of an 'illness of the soul', and as such was the result of a disturbed relationship with those psychic forces that reason could no longer steer. The fact that reason was absent presupposed, in a sense, the incurability of such 'illness', for how could that missing reason ever come back and insert itself once more in order to stem those passions? Indeed, such manifestations of an excess of feeling necessarily resulted in a 'sickness unto death'.

Johann Wolfgang Goethe expressed it most notoriously in his novel of unrequited love, derangement and suicide, *The Sorrows of Young Werther*, published in 1774: "we call it a sickness unto death when nature is so severely attacked and her strength so far exhausted, placed so out of action that she is unable to recover, and no matter what happy change take place is unable to reassert the usual course of life... Observe a man in his natural confined condition; consider how ideas work upon him, and how impressions affect him, till at length a violent passion seizes him, destroys all his powers of calm reflection, and utterly ruins him".

Human nature, according to Goethe's novella, can "endure a certain degree of joy, sorrow and pain, but collapses as soon as this is exceeded". Suicide is an illness and it is, of course, a fatal one: "Nature can find no way out of the labyrinth of confusion and contradiction and so the person must die."

Goethe tells the story of a young man who suffers the extremes of unrequited love and, in the end, takes his own life. The book was a best-seller and became famous as an opportunity for fashionable ladies to read, empathise and weep. "Werther fever" swept Germany and scores of young men dressed up in Werther's garb of yellow waistcoat and blue coat and, like him, shot their brains out.

Moses Mendelssohn's *On Sensitivity* (1755) states that there is no excuse for a rational person to commit suicide. The person who allows the soul to be darkened by passion is to blame for the pain and sadness experienced. C. H. Spiess in his tales of deranged, jilted lovers, *Biographies of the Mad*, writes of each miserable wretch as "the author of his unhappiness."

Likewise, Goethe's heartbroken hero Werther also insists that it is not the world that is responsible for his pain and his drive towards suicide but himself: "I feel only too well that all blame lies with me... in me is concealed the root of all misery." However, in contrast to the prevailing attitude of the time, Goethe's book does not condemn suicide morally. Suicide is associated with heroic deeds, and with the assertion of autonomy. Suicide – brought about by depression – is a contradiction of the Enlightenment belief in the possibility of human perfection and rational social organisation. It is in battle with the very form of reason. Werther opposes a subjective life-principle to bourgeois order. The rhythm of life is the reason of the seasons; true rationality lies within nature, not within the inhuman wheeling and dealing of society. Through Werther, Goethe calls into question the bourgeois ideal of 'reason' or 'rationality', and he investigates the contradictions of individual freedom and conforming to the social order. He illustrates the sensual nature of people, which must go against the categories put forward by the social order. Werther's suicide is inevitable and compulsive and yet, in taking his life, he also asserts his 'self-control' and autonomy – both Enlightenment ideals. He insists upon his rights as he dies with an unlimited self-consciousness and an understanding of his situation. His self-determination consoles him: "however confined he may be he still preserves in his heart the sweet feeling of liberty, and knows that he can leave this prison whenever he likes." The harp player, in another, later work by Goethe, *Wilhelm Meister's Apprenticeship* (1795), carries poison on his person to ensure the same freedom of choice.

Goethe's study of melancholy was a product of the anthropologically-oriented philosophy of the late eighteenth century, in which intellectuals looked hard at their own humanity. For some sections of the intelligentsia, the Enlightenment was seen as a revolution of the self. In Germany, this soul-searching was a by-product of the intellectuals' actual distance from any decisive political power. Goethe had been part of the *Storm and Stress* movement, a grouping of 'angry young men' who became involved in questions of individual psychology. Moritz's journal of experiential psychology (1783-93, Berlin) contained a collection of reports on journeys into the human "inside", to observe psychic curiosities. Doctors, teachers, preachers and others presented countless pathological or psychiatric cases of neurosis, depression and so on. These mental disturbances were then often related back to psychological causes and the suggested cures lay in the realm of psychological treatment and "moral management." Again then the shift from bodily treatment to mental approaches is perceptible. Goethe was a part of this in his search for the inner causes of Werther's melancholy.

The German bourgeois intellectual of the eighteenth century, denied a voice by an oppressive autocratic regime, fell into melancholia. The intellectual turned away from a world that was still effectively in the possession of the nobility. The refuges of bourgeois melancholy lay outside of society, in an appreciation of 'loneliness'. The causes of melancholy were correspondingly positioned within the individual. The tragedy of this melancholia was the ever-narrowing inward journey, where the only destination was the absolute and final removal of the self from the oppressive order. The journey into the self worked upon the self – the ego crumbled, the self dispersed into fragments, impulses, dreams, fantasies (these all found their way into Romantic fiction), and in the end there resulted the absenting of the self from the everyday world, perhaps through death.

This loss of rationality could have had its compensations, ensuring removal from the burden of actuality. Heinrich, the village madman whom Werther encounters, is happiest when completely beyond reason, beside himself: "God in heaven! Is this the destiny of man? To be happy only before he has acquired his reason and again after he has lost it!"

If the only possible strategy of resistance to alienation was self-isolation and a journey into one's own soul, then inside these stony vaults might too have lain the causes and the possibility of a cure. German philosophers and philosophical doctors characterised madness as a form of illness whereby the 'mental' faculties of an ill person fell into disarray and led to obsession with an idée fixe and hallucinations or intense sadness. A prevalent understanding of madness relied upon the conception of the person as outlined in German philosopher Immanuel Kant's writings. Kant insisted that the person was a "free-acting being" or a "self-determining being gifted with reason." Kant postulated that only the subject itself – asserting its reason – could cure its own madness and release itself from "mental immaturity." Only the subject could save itself, and yet, at the same time, only the subject had put itself in such a position.

For Kant there were no causes of madness. Madness was innate and inherited, not elicited by external, social factors. It was the disposition of a person, such as is the case with Werther and another of Goethe's characters, Mad Lila (see *Lila*, reprinted in G. Diener: *Goethe's Lila: Heilung eines Wahnsinns durch psychische Kur*, 1971). Lila is "always too little in her thoughts."

In 1798, Kant wrote: "One often asserts the chance causation of this illness, so that it may be understood not as inherited but acquired, as if the unhappy wretch is himself to blame. "He became mad through love." ...But to fall in love with an inappropriate person with whom any thought of marriage would be the greatest madness, is not the cause but the effect of madness." (*Anthropologie in Pragmatischer Hinsicht*)

The cause was internal; madness, for Kant, was "an inherited disturbance of the mind" and "the outbreak of an unbalanced disposition." 'Mental immaturity' meant an 'understanding' with "weaknesses in respect of its exercise." Reason was absent. These weaknesses existed in women, children and the insane. The mad were excluded from the possibility of ever attaining 'mental maturity': "There is little use in doing anything about it, for it is a case of the powers of the subject not participating (unlike in the case of physical illnesses) and, because only the self-exercise of reason can achieve this goal, all methods of cure must be fruitless in this regard."

This was truly a sickness unto death. Kant continued in his exposition of madness: "The tendency to be turned in on one's self, together with the resulting delusions of the inner senses, can only be brought back into order by leading the person back into the external world and, with that, into the order of things which lies before the external senses." But could this ever be achieved?

Once the exercise of common sense ceased, the subject was no longer a person or moral being. These were identifications that rested on the subject's integration into a community: "The only general characteristic of madness is the loss of a common sense and the logically ensuing singular sense, e.g. in the bright light of day a person sees a burning light on his table, which cannot be seen by another person who is present, or he hears a voice that no-one else can hear. For it is a necessary test of the correctness of our judgements and so too the health of our understanding that we share it with others and are not isolated with our own and yet at the same time judge publicly on the basis of our private ideas."

Now the flaw in Kant's argument becomes apparent. Kant postulated that the subject itself, in a loss of "common sense", produced madness, which was a portrayal of the subjective as objective. This was the 'self-willed mental immaturity', a phrase which implies guilt and immorality. But the origin of madness was also viewed as the effect of a "particular nature", inherited or innate. This would preclude moral criticism.

Somehow Kant maintained that 'unreason' was both produced by the subject and was the innate nature of the subject – it was "blameless blame."

The philosopher Georg Lukács presumed Kant's dilemma was a consequence of the structure of bourgeois society. Here "natural" bonds were being exploded (in the break with the fixed feudal agricultural order) and exchanged for equally rigorous "self-generated" bonds – as in the bourgeois personality who was fixated on accumulation and order. The bourgeois subject was, as the violence against itself necessitated, still an unfree subject. This is the contradiction of bourgeois rule - freedom within constraint - morality and the divinity of money replacing religious edict. The violence of rationality against itself – the Kantian imposition of unfreedom in the act of exercising rationality – was comparable to the status of the mental patient, who was under the rule of an idée fixe. The mental home was the externalised application of 'reason'. Instead of self-administration, it was "being held in order by alien reason." Inside and outside of the mental home, the violence of reason ruled.

MESMERISING DOCTORS

Until the end of the 18th century, the world of the insane was staffed only by the abstract, faceless power that conducted confinement. Then William Tuke, a quaker philanthropist, established a mediating element between guards and patients, between reason and madness, in setting up a retreat in York in 1796. Compassionate moral treatment was the avowed aim. The isolated space of the asylum reserved for insanity was invaded by the prestige of the confining authority, and the vigour of judging reason. 'Self-control' was rewarded and useful occupation encouraged. The 'keeper' now intervened, without violence, instruments of torture or quack treatments; without what in Goethe's play *Lila* is called "dissection, syringing, electrifying." Goethe's play mirrored attempts to find new ways to encounter madness, ways that opened up to delusions, instead of cutting them out. *Lila* used the method of 'psychodrama', allowing the madness to take its place on stage, while the cast/curers find ways to chase out the Mad Lila's illusions, supplanting them gradually with actuality.

The play *Lila* (1777) recounts the story of baroness Lila who is being cured from madness. After she has been mistakenly informed that her husband is dead, she is unable to recognise anybody. When her husband returns, she can no longer recognise him either. Doctor Verazio finds out that she believes her husband to have been imprisoned by evil spirits. These spirits are pursuing her too, and she must find a way to rescue her husband. As part of her cure, Lila has been subjected to brutal measures unsuccessfully. Her doctor says: "I shudder when I think of the cures that have been tried out on her, and I shiver to think of the sort of cruelties that I could have been led to and almost was led to carry out on her."

Under the auspices of this new 'rational' organisation of society, madness was confronted as a being unbalanced, displaced, this being evident in the German word for madness, 'Verrücktheit' – which literally means such displacement. If something or someone had been displaced, knocked off balance, then that individual or thing could be righted again. The mad person could be led back under the guidance of a figure who had been deemed rational. So in Goethe's play there is the idea of Dr. Verazio leading Lila back into the world. Cure here meant leading the figure back from where they had strayed, in order to elicit, ultimately, the desired self-administration.

Dr. Verazio is the figure of rational authority. "With his subtlety", he works without torture or witchcraft, using only his own powerful personality. Dr. Verazio appears as an early psychotherapist, a persuasive patriarch exercising cautious "leading of the soul." This was the scientific age of observation, and of Moritz's "dissection of the soul" and the finding out of individual conditions to enable penetration into the inside, so as to carry out a quite individual course of cure: "the moral doctor must study these illnesses in respect of their appearance, their causes and results, if he intends to cure them."

And yet the violent aspect existed beneath the surface. Dr. Verazio seizes it when it seems necessary. Even in the age of self-declared humanisation of healing, shock treatments were still inflicted. Shock treatment is applied when Lila's dream appears too stubborn and resistant to reason. Fear chases away the fantasy with its concrete brutality. The doctor is prepared to think of the types of violence and injustice that could be used against Lila in order to shake her from her delusion, to knock some sense into her. The threat of a cruel-to-be-kind therapy is never far away.

Dr. Verazio's status as 'priest' is significant. Michel Foucault outlines the new role of the doctor within the asylum in this period: "The doctor's intervention in the asylum is not made by virtue of a medical skill or power that he possesses in himself and that would be justified by a body of objective knowledge. It is not as a scientist that homo medicus has authority in the asylum, but as a wise man." (*Madness And Civilisation*, Tavistock, London, 1971)

The medical profession is here required as a moral and judicial guarantee, rather than as a representative of science. Pinel wrote: "Must it not be an inviolable law in the administration of any establishment for the insane... to grant the maniac all the liberty that the safety of his person and of that of others permits, and to proportion his repression to the greater or lesser seriousness of danger of his deviation... to gather all the facts that can serve to enlighten the physician in treatment, to study with care the particular varieties of behaviour and temperament, and accordingly to use gentleness or firmness, conciliatory terms or the tone of authority and an inflexible severity." In order to treat the patient, the incarcerators must exercise their own judgement, act good cop/bad cop as the situation demands, make decisions rather than incisions..

The idea of a strong personality exerting influence over another person was gaining popularity in medical circles at the time that Goethe wrote *Lila*. In Vienna in 1777, Mesmer healed, at least temporarily, the blind pianist Marie Paradies. This made the 'mesmerist' famous throughout Europe. The woman had already been subjected to leeches, electrification and the like. Mesmer's theory rested on more subtle psychological influences – the gaining of the confidence of the patient and the patient's relations, and the therapeutic use of music. Mesmer saw himself as the mediator of healing. He regarded his therapy as dependent on the benevolent effects of cosmic powers. Magnetism – his healing medium – was seen as a fine, light-like material (materialluminosa) that streamed over the nervous system, healing the mind and the body. This was a combination of modern psychotherapeutic thought, whereby a strong patriarchal figure reinforces authority through his aura, and a metaphysical belief in cosmic power and the healing effects of nature which directly affected the body and soul simultaneously. The physical and psychic are unsplit in this remnant of non-rational, 'scientific' thought.

It is reminiscent of Goethe's understanding of cure in *Lila*. Goethe presents madness, in part, as the possession of the soul by a supernatural thing; an evil spirit, strange powers. The battle is between friendly godheads and the 'demonic'. But in part, Lila's madness is, more conventionally, more modernly, a fault in her capacity to understand rationally, caused by the violent passions unleashed in tragic love. She has lost her mind, her capacity to reason. Drawing on the 18th century idea that violent emotions are illnesses of the mind, by whose appearance 'reason' no longer has control of 'powers of the soul', Goethe shows how the harmonic balance of Lila's inner powers is disturbed and 'apparition' and 'reality' are no longer distinguishable. Lila's cure involves the 'vocal use' of reason. Lila's freedom must come through recognition and labour – the concrete understanding of reality and the self-conscious appropriation of actuality and self. Finally, in the course of cure, fantasy and reality must be made to coincide.

When Lila holds her husband in her arms, having saved him, or rather believing that she has saved him from demons, it is an individual action. She will have got herself to that point, aided by the subtle prompting of Dr. Verazio: "The person helps himself best of all. He must go strolling to find his happiness, he must put his hand out to grab it."

The peculiarity of Dr. Verazio's method is that thereby "one allows the madness to enter, in order to heal the madness." Medics in Goethe's time tended to stress that patients had to be distracted from their fixed delusions. A few medical men had, however, recommended a practice that involved the temporary accessing of the patient's delirium (Johann Christian Reil, Philippe Pinel, Jean-Baptiste Pussin). Reil stated that sometimes, when the cause of madness was not understood, it was "better not to contradict, but to afford belief to his tales" (quoted in G. Diener, *Goethe's Lila*).

The idea of psychodrama – entering the fiction – was an extraordinary procedure. In conventional terms, theatrical representation was a technique opposed to the usual method of awakening of the patient by the labour of reason through slow pedagogy or the imposition through authority. The pact sealed here was a complicity of the unreal with itself: imagination forced to play its own game to cure itself, paradoxically perhaps because there was no obvious dialogue. ("If we could cure fantasy through fantasy" – *Lila*.) If the illusion could appear to be true, then perception could flood the dream, fill in its gaps and integrate the irreality of the image into the perceived truth without one seeming to contradict the other. The role of the priest, the master of ceremonies, was to continue the dialogue of madness in its own language, leading it to convulsion and crisis, whereby the dilemma was confronted by itself and forced to argue against the demands of its own truth.

The priest is compelled to remain within the boundaries of Lila's illusion. It is fortunate that she renounces her belief that her husband is dead, for this then offers the possibility of a dramatic confrontation in her invention of the idea of his imprisonment by demons.

Martin Luther had theorised psychodrama, but it was Reil who made it a practical method, and this was one that was considerably more brutal than the one that Goethe portrayed. On delivery to an asylum, the patient was met with terrifying scenes, drumbeats, cannon fire and thunder. All this was designed to rouse him or her from 'sunkenness into apparition' and compel 'alertness'. Throughout the treatment, dramatic situations were enacted, until finally the patient moved from passive observation of scenes to active participation, to 'self-activity' – the Enlightenment exhortation. The play at the asylum unfolds a shocking theatrical world in which the patient as acting subject must show a willingness to fight with wild animals or demons. The patient is continuously encouraged to new, ever more strenuous, efforts.

Reil called for a grandiose scheme of therapy and organisation of asylums, and psychiatry as an academic discipline. He positioned the doctor at the point where nature fought the distortions of the 'unnatural'. The psychotherapeutic ringmaster was the medium of the nature 'untuned' by the soul; he retuned it.

Battie's influential *Treatise on Madness* (1758) conceived the programme of 'moral management', or the regimentation of madness. This was a steering of the 'mentally ill' linked to the old principle of 'regimen sanitas', necessitating an intimate relationship between doctor and patient. The mediating psychotherapist's role was creative, and his characteristics were those of the artist, Reil maintained. This bears new significance considering that Goethe performed the role of Dr. Verazio when Lila was performed in 1777.

WILHELM MEISTER'S APPRENTICESHIP AND THE RETREAT TO ORDER

A country priest describes the 'assimilation method' of treating the insane in the fifth book of Goethe's *Wilhelm Meister's Apprenticeship*. He says that he finds the methods to cure insanity very simple: "They are precisely the same by which healthy people are prevented from becoming mad. If their spontaneous initiative is aroused, if they are made used to order and if they are given the thought that they share their life and fate with so many others, and that extraordinary talent, the greatest happiness and the most intense misfortunes are only slight deviations from what is usual, then no insanity will creep in, and if it is there it will gradually disappear. I have given the old man a timetable. He teaches the harp to a few children. He helps with work in the garden and is already much more cheerful. He wants to enjoy eating the cabbage that he has planted... As clergyman I try to say only little to him about his strange scruples, but an active life brings with it so many events that he must soon feel that every kind of doubt can only be removed by activity."

The clergyman wants to remove the cowl and beard from the old man, in order to make him the same as the others. Conformity is the cure.

At the close of the 18th century there was general outrage at the incarceration of the insane. Reil spoke of wretches "thrown like state criminals into dungeons where the eye of humanity never penetrates." A new humanitarianism advocated a transposing of the patient into a rural environment where the ordering cycle of daily labour and season changes would restore reason.

The origins of Goethe's harp player's madness lie in unhappy love. It was an incestuous love affair, which unleashed a conflict of conscience. On one level, he is driven insane by the inconceivability of his demanding the right to love in a society which considers incest immoral. On another level, he internalises the guilt that he is made to feel from his transgression: "I have never seen a mind in such an unusual state. For many years he did not make the slightest response to anything outside himself, in fact to anything at all; he merely turned in upon himself, he contemplated his hollow, empty self that seemed to him an immeasurable abyss."

The harp player's madness leaves only the feeling of guilt: "no emotion is left except the feeling of my guilt, which none the less can only be seen in retrospect as a remote, amorphous ghost."

The guilt, which the harp player feels, stems from a strictly upheld taboo on incest, deriving from the church and ignorant of individual desire. The conflict between vital claims and renunciation is unbearable for Augustin. The consciousness of guilt is essentially the cause of the mental disorder.

Sperata, another of Goethe's characters, is also mad due to the guilt imposed by the priest. The priest punishes her for a transgression in the past, but he cannot fully reveal to her what it was that she had done wrong, because he finds the actuality too horrible to admit. He must punish her viciously but she must never know exactly what terrible thing she did: "No sooner had the child been weaned, no sooner did he believe that her body was strong enough to bear the most fearful torment of mind, than he began to paint the transgression to her in terrible colours, the transgression of having yielded to a priest, which he treated as a kind of sin against nature, as a form of incest. For he had the strange idea of making her remorse equal to the remorse she would have felt, if she had learnt about the truth about her misdemeanour."

Goethe demonstrates how the harp player is returned to 'reality' by a therapy that demands self-activity. A desire for order and conformity in an ordered generality is invoked. The country priest expresses his belief in conformity as an essential component of recovery: "for nothing brings us nearer to madness than when we make ourselves different from other people, and nothing preserves our normal reason so much as living in general accord with many people."

The cure is a forcing back into universal bourgeois morality. This is not without some critique of existing social reality. Goethe reproaches the church for its fostering of guilt feelings – both the harp player and Sperata are by nature religiously inclined. And there is a progressive recognition of the social causes of madness: that schooling and civic institutions might play their part in causing it. But what this view omits to mention is that bourgeois normality – an economic system that instituted the slave trade, generated war and imperialism and condemns its populations to soulless drudgery – might itself be mad.

The modern classicist approach saw ideally, in its treatment of madness, chaos dissolved into the wider, ordered universe; the sensuous-empirical and intelligible character of a person brought into an hierarchical order of reason, whereby irrationality was chased out by the internalisation of rationality.

In the early 19th century, ideas of 'fulfilment of duty' began to gain credence in the medical profession. The pedagogic Prussian care method involved an administration of reason and ethical duty, with liberal intent. The aim was an 'internalisation of compulsion'. Curing moved from a mechanical-physical (a knock on the head) to a psychic-moral (a rule in the head) conception. Though Goethe dismissed guilt as a repressive reaction on the part of the clergy, he still understood madness as arising not from a physical or even ultimately social externality, but from within the subject's individual nature. The cure undergone had to be a change in the constitution of the individual who returned – through conformity – to the world of order. The harp player is sent to a retreat to be kept under the watchful eye of the teachings of good sense, truth and morality. The avoidance of physical constraints was part of a system whose essential element was the constitution of self-restraint, made manifest in the submission to labour.

Pinel's retreat was based on the moral power of consolation and a docile obedience to nature. He aimed to resume the moral enterprise of religion, in terms of virtue, labour and social life, and without recourse to the bible. The underlying notion was that, beneath the phenomenon of insanity, the social nature of the essential virtues was not disrupted. At his retreat, Pinel effected moral systems to ensure an ethical continuity between the twin worlds of madness and reason. He constructed an environment which guaranteed bourgeois morality its place as the norm.

Writing of Saragossa, he stated that there had been established "a sort of counterpoise to the mind's extravagances by the attraction and charm inspired by the cultivation of the fields, by the natural instinct that leads man to sow the earth and thus to satisfy his needs by the fruit of his labours. From morning on you can see them... leaving gaily for the various parts of a large enclosure that belongs to the hospital, sharing with a sort of emulation the tasks appropriate to the season, cultivating wheat, vegetables... the surest and most efficacious way to restore man to reason." (quoted in *Madness and Civilisation*)

The changing perception of madness has moved here from the 16th century view of insanity as the product of human animality – a break-out of the primitive nature within – to an understanding of the break with nature as the cause of unreason. This nature, mediated by morality, was now perceived as the very ontological justification and reflection of bourgeois order. Bourgeois order is the natural way, it claims. Liberty in the retreat was put on a level with the laws of nature. The retreat's enforcer of reason bore a different perception of madness to Dr. Verazio. Madness became illusion and as such was cured by the suppression of theatre and artificiality in the return to the illusion-free world of labour. Life in the asylum was essentially a microcosm of bourgeois society and its values.

Psychology itself is in question in *Wilhelm Meisters Apprenticeship*. Wilhelm must learn the pitfalls of introspection, self-analysis and diary-keeping. The journey, the external movement is the 'true' way to discover the self, through social interaction. The heroics of Werther's suicide are no longer relevant. It is the drive to conform, to accept the necessary and control the co-incidental.

Wilhelm is instructed: "The texture of this world is made of necessity and chance; man's reason comes between the two and can dominate them. It treats necessity as the basis of existence, and it can steer, lead and make use of chance factors. Only when it stands firm and unshakeable does man deserve to be called a god of the earth. Unhappy is he who from early age becomes accustomed to trying to find something arbitrary in what is necessary, who would like to attribute to chance elements a kind of reason, the following of which would in fact itself be a matter of religion."

The Kantian model entails a setting of limits on the urge towards freedom: "A person is not happy until his unrestricted striving determines for itself its own limits."

The weakness of the characters in *Wilhelm Meister's Apprenticeship*: the harp player, Mignon, Sperata, the Countess and Aurelie, is that they have not successfully integrated themselves into the objective world by imposing certain limits upon their perceptions of reality. They withdraw into hallucinatory fantasies. The harp player's deluded conviction that he will injure and be injured by a young boy is ultimately more powerful than the healing nature of ordered activities. Nothing can dispel the Count's premonition that he is to die, nor the Countess's belief that the physical imprint of her husband's medallion has caused her to contract cancer. These fixations arise, on the one hand, because of a nature predisposed to effusion and rapture, and on the other, because of a lack of activity and distraction in the external world.

The doctor in *Wilhelm Meister's Apprenticeship* says: "It is a misfortune for anyone to get fixed in his mind some idea or other which has no influence on active life, or even withdraws him from active life."

The notion of a lack of activity causing mental instability is repeated in the sequel, *Wilhelm Meister's Wandering Years* (1821). Leonardo is haunted by the memory of a scene in which "whenever I was alone, whenever I was unoccupied, that image emerged before my soul. It was an insoluble impression, which could be overshadowed by other images and sympathies, but could never be completely purged."

In this context, it is revealing to contrast young Goethe's compassion for Werther with his later assessment of Werther's psychoses in his autobiography *Poetry and Truth* (published in four parts, 1811-1833): "Suicide is a phenomenon of human nature that demands everyone's attention and needs reassessment in every epoch, however much it may already have been discussed and treated. Montesquieu grants his heroes and great men the right to take their lives at will, saying that everyone must be at liberty to conclude the fifth act of his tragedy as he pleases. Moreover, my subject here is not those who have led a significant and active life, who have dedicated their days to some great realm or to the cause of freedom. When the idea that inspired such people has vanished from the earth, we do not begrudge them the wish to carry it into the other world. Here we are concerned with those who actually become disgusted with life because – out of a lack of deeds – they have placed exaggerated demands on themselves in the most peaceful situation imaginable." This is reproach and it insists that there are the little people who are nobodies. Its answer to depression is 'get back to work'.

Werther's melancholy and suicide are seen as caused by a lack of occupation and a youthful error. These were the thoughts of an old, complacent man, who had found a place in the new bourgeois world – he was by now a Prussian bureaucrat and had been admitted to the ranks of the aristocracy - becoming von Goethe - and he no longer understood rebellion. The harmonic synthesis after which Wilhelm Meister must strive is outlined in Goethe's *Maxims and Reflections:* "The botanists have a type of plant that they call incompletae; one can also say that there are incomplete, unfinished people. It is those whose longing and striving is not in proportion with their activity and achievement."

THE REORGANISATION OF MADNESS

In the Middle Ages, madness was associated with forbidden knowledge of the Fall and with the divine madness of Christ's redemption. During the classical Enlightenment period, madness came to be perceived as a violation of the orderly and rational laws of nature. It is telling that beggars and criminals were not seen to have transgressed reason, but rather the norms of society, and so they could often be immediately reintegrated into the labour market usefully. Anyway, the need for a large subsistence level workforce allowed for social reintegration of the dispossessed – the poor were forced to work. But the mad had to be put away. They could not work, because they were said to possess 'no reason'. They had to be brought back into labour. A moral stigma afflicted the insane, who were to be punished for not conforming to the orderly laws of nature.

Foucault has been influential in detailing the forms of madness over the last half-millennium. He pinpoints three stages of punishment-treatment of deviance in the development of western civilisation: firstly, the 'monarchical', in which punishment is 'technical', that is, a visible attack on the body using torture; secondly, the 'law of the reforming jurists', a 'corrective' practice whereby, in Hegelian terms, the criminal or insane person re-qualifies as a juridical subject by self-willed punishment; thirdly, the 'disciplinal', which involves the normalisation of individuals, understood as the training and mastering of the body, the reintegration into bourgeois morality, through discipline and the making-conscious of individual guilt.

Goethe, a truly knowledgeable individual, fascinated by biology and anthropology, had contact with medical theorists and practitioners throughout his life. Many of Goethe's medical acquaintances, including his alchemist doctor, J.E. Metz, had studied at Halle, where a tradition of 'universal psychiatry' set out from the premise of the superiority of the soul as determinant of good or ill health. Goethe would have been involved in discussions of madness, its apparent composition and supposed causes.

In this epoch, traditional understandings of madness based on the effects of the four humours were in turmoil and subject to revision and debate. From time to time in Goethe's writings, a person diagnosed as mad appears, signalling a certain attitude, on the author's part, to insanity. Goethe's understanding of madness and the possibility of cure shifts as the debates on madness reshape through an age of change. In his plays, novels and scientific writings there is a movement from a championship of madness as emancipation to an increasing burdening of guilt and moral compulsion on the lunatic. Madness came to be pushed out of the harmonic cosmos, rearing its head perhaps only as the symbol of artistic intoxication, not a real madness but the symbol of genial manifestation, which compels to create. Madness and melancholia became, for the mature Goethe, manifestations of an inactive self. Inactivity is an unacceptable attitude in bourgeois society. Madness turns out to be an affront to, and dialectical opposite of bourgeois order.

The question remains: what traces can be found of all this in contemporary psychiatric methods and theories of remedial treatment: occupational therapy, drugs, lobotomies, ECT, 'talking cures', 'care in the community', sections? One thing is certain, madness has a history. Its history inflects in tandem with the needs of the powerful. Madness is the rulebook's cracked mirror. Sometimes madness has an affinity with freedom, with rejection of the norms of society, its constrictions and codes of conduct. Freedom was the Great Idea of a revolutionary bourgeois class. The philosophers and the literati and the politicians exalted freedom, in the name of shattering aristocratic rule. But as they rolled back their own revolution, liberty remained only as an empty phrase, partial and tangled in contradiction. Instead of universal freedom, universal conformity became the rule. The mad must still insist on that freedom, and find ways of grabbing it.

TURNING THE ASYLUM INTO A PLAYGROUND

ROBERT DELLAR

If surveillance techniques work nicely, people and events can be comprehensively observed and controlled in institutions. I once worked in a psychiatric hospital at a time when its surveillance techniques weren't working too well.

The Hackney Hospital was located in Homerton - one of the most deprived parts of Western Europe and rough even by Hackney standards. Over the years, Homerton had become a psychiatric ghetto. Most of the borough's in-patient and community mental health services came to be based there, along with drug clinics, residential units and the notorious sink estate called the Kingsmead. These days, a walk along Homerton High Street takes you past very few pedestrians who haven't used psychiatric services. The district's reputation as a dustbin for nutters isn't new, though; it has had a long history of development.

Hackney Poor House opened its doors in the High Street in 1729, housing 15 local paupers. It moved across the road in 1741 to a bigger building where there were 30 paupers. By 1764, the number of paupers had increased to 48, spread across a total of five rooms. Various huts and sheds were annexed; by 1834 the already high local level of deprivation had been worsened by epidemics of cholera and smallpox, and no fewer than 380 of Hackney's poor lived in the complex. It goes without saying that many of these people were mad.

After 1841 the institution was revamped and new buildings were erected - buildings which were inhabited right up until Hackney Hospital's closure in 1995. The new set-up was a Victorian workhouse with as many as 1,030 inmates by 1930, plus an additional 663 people who were medically monitored in the workhouse infirmary. From 1930, the institution stopped being a workhouse and was re-classified as a hospital. At first it housed a wide range of medical disciplines, but by the time I arrived in 1992 the place was being run down. Many of the buildings had already been abandoned; the only inmates left were mad ones.

With the gradual evacuation of the buildings came a decrease in numbers of staff keeping an eye on the site. This made it easier for people to cause trouble. For example, soon after I began work I heard about some tramps who had managed to find an entrance to the basement beneath the block containing most of the acute psychiatric wards. The tramps had lived there for a while, burning old piles of forgotten medical records to keep themselves warm and so that they could see. They were evicted only when a newspaper ran an article after getting wind of the occupation from a Kingsmead resident who was notorious for his money-making scams and for drunkenly chasing children around the forecourts of the estate armed with a machete. Though such behaviour is by no means unusual on the Kingsmead, some people regarded his testimony as unreliable.

By 1992 the hospital was falling to bits. It really was a tip: even one of the psychiatrists described it in the local rag as a 'rat-pit'. It was ripe for demolition, and needed to be replaced by a supermarket. Homerton is poorly served for decent supermarkets. The nearest is Tescos in Well Street, nearly a mile away, and even this is very small in comparison with the larger branches of Tescos near to Seven Sisters and Bethnal Green tube stations. It amazes me that, as I write, the empty and rotting blocks still haven't been knocked down, when clearly they should make way for a large branch of Sainsburys.

The last years of the hospital saw frequent burst sewage pipes which led to floods of human waste from the upper floors engulfing the lower parts of the building. By this time the heating system had two settings - on, and off. Usually it was on, causing the block and everyone inside to melt in stifling, oppressive heat. The whole place was collapsing, but there were unusual opportunities for fun and games which did a little, if nowhere near enough to counter the negative vibrations and bad karma accumulated over long, tragic years of boredom, torture and incarceration.

When they weren't sheltering tramps, the empty spaces allowed arts projects to take root. Core Arts, a progressive mental health group, began when local artist Paul Monks used an abandoned ward as a studio. A few patients stumbled across him accidentally, and he allowed them to use his materials to make their own work. Things snowballed, and within a few weeks dozens of mad artists were discovering their creativity. Funding was secured, a recording studio was added, and Core Arts went on to find its own premises and go from strength to strength. Quite separately, an art exhibition - 'Rear Window' - took shape across the hospital grounds as they were cleared, and works by famous names like Derek Jarman co-existed with pieces by many local survivor artists. These initiatives deservedly met with widespread acclaim, unlike some of the other things going on at the same time.

In 1994 I helped set up Hackney Patients Council, a kind of union: in spite of its beginnings, the Council is now a respectable organisation taken seriously by professionals. While the hospital slowly ground to a halt, a plan for the Council's launch party was hatched in the advocacy office on the ground floor of F block, beneath the acute wards. For a start, we ordered some food, bought a load of fireworks and made several trips to the off licence to stock up on booze. Also we were lucky to be in contact with top sculptor Keith "Mally" Mallinson, who took advantage of F block's lax security to climb the stairs to Connolly Ward on the top floor, where he discreetly observed Dr. Trevor Turner, the controversial consultant psychiatrist for the south east quarter of Hackney, showing the junior shrinks how it was done in his ward round. Mally got out his note pad and sketched a reasonable likeness of the doctor.

On the day of the party, Mally and his assistant Earil Hunter, formerly of the British karate team, gathered a collection of wooden pallets and other stuff from the site of the medium secure unit being built nearby. A tall pile of inflammable material grew outside the nurses' home, a building on the hospital grounds still occupied by poorly paid nurses living in box rooms. Meanwhile the advocacy office and adjacent disused rooms, previously ECT suites, began to teem with current and former patients. It was November the fifth.

Nearly all of the in-patients who were allowed out unescorted had turned up, and they were knocking back the abundant supply of beer and wine. Animated chatter competed for audibility with the ghetto blaster pounding out reggae and soul. Surprisingly this went on for some hours unchallenged by hospital staff, despite a few curious nurses wandering in and helping themselves to the booze, asking us not to grass them up to the ward managers for drinking on the job. You would have assumed that it was a normal house party, if it wasn't for the fact that many of the patients wore hospital pyjamas.

The party wore on, the booze kicked in, and two impressive artworks were unveiled. The first was a tall, colourful portrait of Dr. Turner, painted with oils by Jill Cleghorn. The masterpiece, entitled 'The Doctor of My Dreams', depicted the shrink naked except for stockings and suspenders. Next, Mally's creation was revealed: sat on a chair, the Patients Council 'guy', a life-size and remarkably accurate effigy of Dr. Turner made out of papier mache and other materials, complete with suit, tie, spectacles and clinical gaze checking for symptoms.

Unfortunately, the hospital site co-ordinator found out about the wooden heap that had appeared outside the nurses' home and she made several frantic and concerned telephone calls to the advocacy office while the party was in full swing. For some reason, she had this idea that we were planning a bonfire later. After being threatened with the police we backed down, but a compromise was reached and we were permitted to set off our fireworks.

Outside, darkness drew in early, and reports reached the party of drunken, disorderly behaviour from the wards above. One or two patients had puked and the nurses had had to clear it up. Also many were being unusually boisterous and giving the nurses a hard time. Several bottles of wine had been confiscated.

Leaving Trevor on his chair, we announced that the party was moving to the tarmac outside the nurses home. The pyre was still there but would remain unlit, giving the effigy a reprieve. In the small garden area next to the staff residential quarters, fresh fireworks were planted: no expense had been spared and most of them were more than a foot long. Showers of stars and sparks in glorious rainbow colours cascaded into the sky above as a succession of roman candles, catherine wheels and fizzy volcanoes held the audience's attention. One or two nurses came out to watch but behaved themselves and didn't interfere.

Each firework seemed somehow bigger than the one before, and in our growing excitement we set off more and more of them in one go each time. Snaps, crackles and pops thundered loudly, defiant and somehow eerie, across the hospital grounds, fierce explosions echoing and ricocheting against the nineteenth century buildings. Finally, we were down to the last firework - a rocket, which was nearly seven feet long, including its stalk!

We didn't have a milk bottle big enough to launch it from, but eventually we found a suitable litter bin. Mally lit the touchpaper and we all stood back. Hushed expectancy mingled with trepidation: it was the biggest firework any of us had ever seen!

After what seemed like ages the rocket took off and flew gloriously into space, sparkling and shining like the brightest shooting star before reaching its climax: a nuclear explosion, multi-coloured sheets of lightning turning the sky from dark to light for miles around. Chaos escalated and there were scenes unwitnessed in East London since the blitz. Throughout the square half-mile of the hospital grounds, from each wall of every building, bright, blinding bulbs flashed wildly: brilliant, high-powered lights we hadn't known were there. It wasn't dark anymore: in fact, the deranged glare was completely overwhelming. At the same time, an air raid siren pierced the atmosphere at a volume of hundreds of decibels, its source seemingly from every molecule of matter in the grounds; deafening and ghastly. Those of us loosely responsible for 'organising' the party decided it was time to make ourselves scarce and go to the pub. Rushing back to where the party had been to collect our belongings, we encountered a gang of domestics and nurses stampeding down the stairs in panic like demented pigs.

"They're smoking dope in the toilets, that's what's set the fire alarm off!" shouted one nurse. She was annoyed.

"They're drunk, all of them!" complained another nurse who wasn't too pleased either.

Trying to look innocent we got our stuff and left, in time to witness a dozen fire engines all speeding into the hospital grounds. We had a fair-sized crew, and there was a punk nite at the late-opening tavern the Jolly Butchers in Stoke Newington, so we flagged down some taxis and went. Most of us were slaughtered already, but carried on drinking as we gloated over the day's achievements until chucking out time came at one o'clock in the morning.

As we staggered onto the pavement, a police van approached and slowed down. The cops inside glared at us menacingly; we responded with a volley of V-signs and shouts of "wankers!" and "cunts!" The van stopped, a cop jumped out and randomly grabbed a character named Rob Colson, slamming him up against the wall. Mally dragged the pig away and smacked him in the mouth. The other cops jumped out of the van like the SAS storming into action, pushing Mally to the ground and kicking him about viciously. From his prone position Mally managed to give as good as he got, getting in a fair few kicks and punches before grabbing hold of a copper's bollocks, squeezing hard and pulling brutally. The rest of us tried to break it up but the street fight was all over very quickly, and within seconds Rob, Mally and a Japanese bloke walking past at the time and nothing to do with it were bundled into the back of the meat wagon which sped away, leaving the rest of us there shell-shocked. Mally was given a good kicking in the van on the way to the station. He tried to roll under the seats but the cops kept dragging him out. By the time he, Rob and the tourist were charged the next morning with assaulting police officers and resisting arrest, he was black and blue. Rob was also done for possession of speed, but the charges were later dropped. Sadly, it turned out that the Japanese guy went on to kill himself.

The effigy sat in the advocacy office for a fortnight until an arrangement was made to burn him in a neighbour's back garden. Dr. Turner was thrown onto the grass, petrol was sprayed all over him and then the bastard was set alight. Watching the establishment pillar and controversial authority figure go up in flames was a truly moving and heart-warming experience for the several dozen spectators. A number of bangers and fireworks had been inserted into the psychiatrist's body, and they exploded in fits and starts as the cremation took its course. The doctor's bones weren't made out of any old rubbish, they were good quality stuff: firm, solid wood that combusted at its own pace without losing any spectacular effect. The wood had been sculpted into the exact shape of a human skeleton, and as the flesh began to melt and drip away, a perfect bone structure was revealed and glowed a pleasant shade of red as the doctor decomposed; the rib-cage was particularly splendid. The event became an occult ceremony: several spectators pissed ritually over the embers and some hocus-pocus was uttered. We imagined that the real doctor would fail to appear at work the following day. Finally the fire burnt out and all that was left of the eminent professional was the lower part of one of his legs, still wearing a smart and polished shoe.

After this, Dave Fanning from punk band the Apostles produced a chinese firecracker incorporating no fewer than 750 bangers, including some huge ones nearly as large as the missile that had struck the hospital barely two weeks earlier. There were children's swings at the end of the garden and Dave attached the firecracker cautiously to the frame. Making sure that the crowd stood well back, Dave held his lighter at arm's length, lit the touchpaper and ran like fuck. There was a lengthy succession of ever-loudening explosions as the flame manoeuvred its way around the maze of fuse: thundering and cacophonous, the sound of the sky itself crashing to the ground: the apocalypse!

As soon as the sonic attack ceased, frenzied shouting erupted across the neighbourhood and the people in the flats opposite peered, afraid, from behind their net curtains. And then the sirens: police cars, ambulances, fire engines - the lot. Surprisingly they pulled up outside a house down the road and it was several minutes before they picked on us. We pretended to be sensible. It transpired that the vibrations caused by the giant firecracker had caused the roof of the nearby house to collapse. Somehow we fronted it out, but the tradition of inviting public services along to Patients Council events was now firmly established.

The hospital was still open but winding down fast. Exploring the corridors, wards and offices of the now deserted G and H blocks was an interesting pursuit. The place hadn't been colonised by junkies: the syringes scattered liberally across the floors had all been left behind by the medical staff. There were rubber gloves, medical records, ECT machines, desks, tables, filing cabinets, iron lungs, scalpels, stethoscopes, straightjackets and all sorts of other paraphernalia: a treasure-trove of medical waste. Heartbreakingly, one of the empty wards, a psychogeriatric unit, was filled to the ceiling with forgotten paintings representing perhaps the final testaments of their creators, discarded and dumped just as the painters and their predecessors had been discarded and dumped into the Hackney Hospital. Faces, landscapes and abstract images, some unbelievably bleak, all destined to be crushed beneath the bulldozers along with the hollow tombstone in which they lay abandoned.

And yet the building remained overdue for demolition. It should have been knocked down years previously. I managed to salvage a few of the paintings, but sadly I lost them somewhere along the line.

Other events during this period included punk concerts, poetry nights and football matches organised by the Patients Council. Finally, 266 years after Hackney Poor House first opened, the institution reached its last night and a party was thrown to celebrate. It was co-organised by the Council and 'Rainbow' ward staff in order to usher in a new spirit of co-operation, but sadly this attempted partnership failed as the senior Rainbow nurse became distressed by Council members' drinking and bad language. Using her walkie-talkie, the nurse 'bleeped' her immediate senior, a ward manager once alleged to have restrained a patient who was eight months pregnant by sitting on her stomach. He was pleased to spoil the fun by bringing the party to a premature end.

Questions were asked later. Whenever a Patients Council event took place at the hospital, staff, especially middle management, always wanted to know who was in charge. They'd been indoctrinated so thoroughly with the hierarchy structure of nursing that they thought it inconceivable that anything could function otherwise. "Nobody's in charge, we all take responsibility" we told them. "I'm sorry," a baffled nursing manager replied, "I don't get you..."

It had been talked about and delayed for so long that nobody thought it would ever really happen. But one day F block had four wards full of patients, and the next, everyone was gone and the hospital grounds were deserted save for a few security guards and hangers-on from the arts projects mentioned earlier. A lot of equipment was left behind, and I managed to scavenge a fridge from one of the empty wards. I'd destroyed my previous one on the same day, trying to defrost it by scraping at the freezer compartment with a knife. I'd never thought about how fridges worked, and it was a surprise when toxic gas started to hiss from the wound my blade had cut into the lining. Some of the other workers at the hospital also ended up with fridges and other household items.

They'd built another hospital around the corner. It was exactly the same as the old one, only newer and more efficient. There were now very few holes in the institutional armour, and spy cameras were everywhere. For a few days after it opened, the security staff couldn't stop looking at the monitors in their office. They couldn't believe it: all that vision and power. They were charging round the unit reacting to the slightest hint of misdemeanour, challenging people urinating in the corridors or smoking in the wrong place. And then the novelty wore off and things settled down. It's not the kind of place where you can get away with fireworks or wacky arts projects, but the institutional gaze has its blind spots. At the ends of some corridors there are corners that the cameras can't see. Small parties take place in these corners, and the cleaners have to sweep away the joint butts and empty beer cans daily.

ESCAPE FROM THE EDGE
EDWARD MURRAY

I was born at home on 26th July 1959 at Drumlodge Drumany, Letterkenny, Co. Donegal. I had always believed that I was the heaviest baby in our family as my mother had told me that I had weighed over 10lbs. It was only when I was first admitted to a mental hospital that my sister made me aware of the fact that I had been born prematurely, and had won a hard fight for survival. Obviously my mother hadn't wanted to give me an inferiority complex. This had worked.

My earliest memory is of my first day at school. My mother and another mother arranged for their sons' first day there to coincide with a party for the children receiving Holy Communion for the first time. Our teacher was a great woman, a real Prime-of-Miss-Jean-Brodie type. When I was about five we had a slight altercation. I had been naughty, and she called me to the front of the class for four slaps on the hand with a sally rod. I took my punishment bravely and walked back to my seat smiling to my friends, so she said to me that obviously that hadn't been enough for me and to come back up for another four. I went back up, but when she struck me again I closed my tiny fist around the cane. I pulled it from her hand and proceeded to break it into a dozen pieces, after which I told her that I'd had my punishment, miss, and how I take it is my business. Then I walked back to my seat and tears began to well up in my eyes. I was so proud of my little stand for justice. I don't recall her ever hitting me again.

My disenchantment with the Catholic religion also began at about this time. I remember being taught about Adam and Eve in Catechism class, and I asked the teacher who did Cain and Abel marry. She told me not to ask stupid questions. Well, I thought (although not in the vernacular): this is a load of bollocks.

My disillusionment with the church grew much deeper and even to the point of bitterness whilst I was in my teens, when I realised that it was due to the church's inaction and lack of leadership that Britain had managed to occupy Ireland for so long. Let me explain: when Catholicism was persecuted in Ireland under the penal laws, the first of which was enacted in 1697, the seminaries came from France filled with ideas of revolution. This proved a real thorn in Britain's side, and so Britain came up with the idea of building Maynooth college in 1795. It was for the training of Catholic priests in Ireland and with the implicit understanding that if you scratch my back, I'll scratch yours: and so they divided up the country between them.

I also came to believe in the ordination of women, the abolition of the rules on celibacy within the priesthood, contraception, sex before marriage, homosexual rights and divorce, and the right of a woman to have an epidural during childbirth: this was opposed by the church because the Bible says that from the screaming and wailing of woman, Man is born.

Although my father was a farmer, I realised pretty early on that the land wasn't going to be for me. One Christmas I got a toy tractor for a present and I loved it, and so I asked for the same thing the following Christmas. When I got a spinning top I realised straight away that the land was for one of my older brothers.

I left school at fourteen years of age, after one year of college. I wanted to smoke and drink and be out chasing girls, so I got a job in a bakery. I was the head baker by the time that I was sixteen, with about ten men under me. However, although I was doing a man's work, the boss there thought that he could get away with paying me a boy's wage and so I left that job before I turned seventeen. I got work as a fitter's mate on a big construction site, where I told them that I was eighteen, so I could get the man's wage. After that job finished, I came to England for the first time, to Preston in Lancashire, when I was about nineteen, with two friends to work as labourers on various building sites. This work did not impress me. When I returned to Ireland at Christmas, after four months away, I vowed that I would at least have a trade if I was ever to go back there again.

After Christmas I signed up for a welding course at ANCO. I completed this five months later, and got a job at an engineering firm in Lifford. After nine months there I was promoted to foreman of fabrication and welding, but unfortunately due to bad management the company went bust a little over a year later. I then did an advanced welding course as an ASME IX pipe welder. From this I got work on one of the biggest construction programmes in Europe, the Alcan Aughanish Island Project. Near to the end of this job I met my first real love and I decided to go and live in Donegal again; but work prospects were not great there. I had to take a job at an engineering firm, doing work for which I was actually overqualified.

After about two years at this place I suffered a minor injury, a broken foot, and we fell out over compensation. I found myself unemployed for the first time, and without any real prospects. The strain of all this led to depression and my abundance of confidence disappeared. My relationship with my fiancée deteriorated and we eventually broke up. And so, after a few months of being a virtual recluse, I decided to come to England for a second time, this time to London. I had about £150 in my pocket, but a friend who had been in the capital before clued me up on how to get accommodation from the DHSS. I booked immediately into a B&B in Victoria and I took my bill along to the local social security office. I came out of there with about £140 and I thought, this is a great country!

I booked into a hostel in Kensington. I deliberately did not go to an Irish area for two reasons: firstly because I wanted to work at my trade as a welder and metal worker, and secondly because I wanted to preach the gospel of Irish Republicanism according to Eddie Murray.

I got an opportunity to do this very quickly, as on my first night out in central London I met with three young soldiers who were about to be posted to Northern Ireland within the next few days. We talked all night about what lay ahead of them and about the history of the conflict between Britain and Ireland. I was appalled to learn that they were taught that every Catholic was a possible enemy while every Protestant was a possible friend. I then realised that it was clearly a job for the United Nations. Still, I can only say that I hope they were better soldiers for having met me, and that they all returned home safely.

As I have mentioned my gospel of Irish Republicanism, let me explain just what that is. I can understand why Lloyd George insisted on the partition of Northern Ireland back in 1920. After all, Britain had just finished the Great War with Germany and the possibility of an independent Ireland becoming an ally of France, Germany or even Russia and allowing them to land in Ireland and attack Britain through its back door, that must have struck fear into its leaders. They decided that they had to keep a foothold in Ireland so that they could deploy their troops quickly to counter any threat: even though it meant the partition of the province of Ulster as well as the island of Ireland and the installation of the minority as a majority. After the Second World War, Northern Ireland became strategically important as the cold war intensified. It was a launching point, an observation post for the Atlantic Ocean. The sad thing is that the Unionists understood exactly the position that they were in and saw it as a carte blanche to set up a virtual apartheid state. And so it went on for fifty years, the Unionists safe in the knowledge that Britain could not object to how they were conducting their affairs. Until 1969, when the civil rights movement appeared, beaten into existence. The Unionists burned out Catholics in their hundreds. I was only ten years old but I remember the refugee camps along the Donegal border.

But on with my story: after about three weeks I got a job as a welder-metalworker at a company that made TV scenery for the BBC. It was well paid and interesting work and I learned new skills quickly, like using a calculator for doing my trigonometry. Back in Donegal we had worked out angles by drawing everything out on the floor, which took up space, and was time-consuming and less accurate.

However, although it was a great job, with hindsight I was leaving myself wide open to paranoia because of my overt political stance.

Within a year I was a bit of a wreck and taking time off sick. I would imagine that my fellow work-mates were drugging me with cannabis, speed or even acid in my coffee, and I would break out in cold sweats and generally feel as if I was going mad.

In October 1985, after about a year in that job, I was referred to a psychiatrist for the first time. At my first appointment she asked me what the problem was but I couldn't tell her, and instead just broke down in tears. At the next appointment she had a student in with her to observe me and I thought, I'm not going to give a repeat performance of the last time. When she asked what was wrong, I said that basically I needed to get my act together. Unfortunately English was not her first language and she didn't understand the expression. 'What do you mean, get my act together?' she asked, as if I were some type of a showman or something. So I thought, 'this is a waste of time'. I left, telling her that I didn't want any further appointments.

Although I loved my job and it was rather a thrill seeing our work on television, everything from *Top Of The Pops* and *Doctor Who* to *Mastermind* and many more, I quit that Christmas and got work welding on building sites. My paranoia greatly decreased as I was working mainly with other Irish people and I didn't feel the same pressure. My confidence, however, was still low and my love life was not great; I was living with a girl I did not love, and we broke up after about six months. For the next four years I worked on various sites and workshops, all less prestigious and less well paid than the BBC job but they caused less paranoia. In March 1989 I found myself in a room in Southall working in a workshop that made tipper trailers.

I had moved into the room about two weeks beforehand and had not been in contact with my family to tell them my new address. I was watching the BBC nine o'clock news one Friday evening and I saw a report on an accident in Northern Ireland. A woman's car had stalled on a railway crossing, and she had been killed and her children injured. The report showed where it had happened and the wreckage of the car. I knew it was a crossing that my sister used and that her car was a Fiesta and I went into shock, fearing the worst. About two hours later I eventually gathered the courage to 'phone my brother-in-law. When he answered the 'phone we talked amicably for about two minutes and then he said, 'is there a reason why you phoned?' and I told him what it was. He said, 'I'm afraid it was Annie'. I just dropped the 'phone and punched the place to pieces. My beloved sister, the most successful member of the family with a PhD in science, was dead. I managed to scrape enough money together and borrow some clean clothes, suitable for a funeral, and I made my way home. This was a real transition point in my life. I thought how could I best

honour my sister's memory, and I decided to really go for my
ambitions and seek to fulfil my potential as she would have wanted.

When I returned to London I immediately enrolled on an Access to Science
course. I wanted to broaden my education as much as possible, although my
real ambitions lay in Law and Politics. I was really focused for the next year
and did not suffer too much from paranoia. I won a place at the London
School of Economics and Political Science, after an interview, an entrance
exam and passing the access course with a distinction. The paranoia really
started again when I started to do Law at the LSE; but there's a saying, 'just
because you're paranoid it doesn't mean they're not out to get you'.
Especially after the IRA bombings, I would overhear people saying 'look at
that wanker' and various other things behind my back. I began to imagine a
vast conspiracy against me, which wasn't helped by incidents such as one
lecturer, Ewan McKendrick, telling anti-Irish jokes during a lecture. I began
to lose all faith in the impartiality of the LSE and then I started to have
hallucinations. I remember once watching television late at night in the halls
of residence TV room, and the television started to do double-takes and I
thought, 'they are damned clever, this bunch of conspirators against me'.

I also started to get paranoid amongst the Irish community at this time. I
thought that they must have thought me a traitor to the cause because I was
studying Law at an English university. Also I had been along to a Dave Allen
concert in the Strand. I was sitting in the balcony and I thought that his entire
show consisted of jokes at my expense. I felt like jumping off, but I didn't
want to hurt anybody down below. This is where my feelings of alienation
from the Irish people began. All along I thought that the conspiracy against
me involved a vast underground betting syndicate, who were gambling on
how I would react next. I went on a visit to Oxford University to see a
girlfriend I had met in Germany. She wasn't there and as I was leaving
Oxford I looked up at a billboard hoarding and saw an advertisement for a
film, 'The Lion comes to Oxford but doesn't score'. I got dressed up in my
best suit and went down to the Albert Hall to fight Frank Bruno, easily
gaining entry although I did not have a ticket. I remember saying to the
usherette, 'is Frank here yet?' but then a piano-playing comedian came on
and, like Dave Allen, began telling jokes about me. After the interval I got up
on stage and started to play the piano. I was restrained and thrown out.

In the summer, after my first year exams, which I managed to scrape
through with a 2:2, I got a job on a welding contract in Bonn in Germany. I
was on about £400 a week but I was so untogether by now that I only
managed to hold it down for about two weeks before being sacked for the
first time in my life. I had a few quid, so I dumped my tools and
decided to go travelling through Europe. I made my way by hitching

lifts and organising rides through the Mitfahrzentrale down to Geneva in Switzerland, where I met some people and was invited to stay at this wonderful old mansion squat. One of the inhabitants there had a guitar and when he heard me play and sing Irish folk songs he suggested that I try busking, which I did. I found it both very lucrative and a great way to meet people. After spending three weeks there I decided to go to Lyon in France. I bought my own guitar and spent the rest of the summer having a wonderful time with many girlfriends, travelling around France and Spain.

I returned refreshed to meet my second year at the LSE, but my confidence in the impartiality of the establishment was never really restored and the paranoia quickly returned. I did not endear myself to the Tory students during this second year. They had invited Edwina Currie to speak and, as it was the time of the Gulf War, she went on about how proud she was to be British in this moment. I stood up and said to her, 'Ms. Currie, I don't know how you travelled here today but you must have come one of three ways, either down the Strand, down Kingsway or up Fleet Street, but whichever way you came you would have had to have been blind not to have noticed the people living in shop doorways in cardboard boxes'. I asked her whether she felt proud to be British when she noticed these scenes. I also attacked Peter Brook, the Northern Ireland secretary when he came to speak, a man whom I had previously admired for his efforts in the province. However, he gave a very partisan and patronising speech and I got up and I very angrily called him a cunt, and said that he was talking like somebody who wanted to make a silk purse from a sow's ear.

I had no girlfriend at this time and my social life was not great either, and the hallucinations increased. My ambition was to be a barrister and I was still handing in the work, but then I discovered that a life at the bar entailed swearing an oath of allegiance to the Queen. This ruined it for me and I became quite directionless, although I managed to complete the year with another 2:2. Once again I went back to the welding during the summer holidays, in a workshop in Hayes, Middlesex, where I had worked before starting university. I saved some money and decided to travel through the United States. I planned to busk my way around.

However, America wasn't set up for busking in quite the same way as Europe with its outside café seating arrangements. Although I saw New York, Boston, Baltimore, Ocean City and Philadelphia, money started running out fast. I had to return to London, where I drew on my overdraft and travelled over to Amsterdam. It didn't prove lucrative, however, and I was getting deeper into debt. I returned to face my final year at the LSE with an element of dread, but determination in my heart.

My third year was dreadful; I got a room with an alcoholic in a high-rise near Euston and, after a few months there and several political discussions, I was attacked one night, leaving me with twenty-five stitches to the head. I moved out of there into a horrible bedsit in Earl's Court.

The hallucinations and the paranoia got really terrible. The hallucinations were visual as well as auditory. I remember watching 'Star Trek' and Captain Kirk was talking to Uhuru and he said, 'this will get the whore'. Now I know that this was an hallucination, but at the time his lip movements matched exactly what I had heard him say. It never occurred to me that I was going crazy. I just thought how clever the conspirators were. I started hearing personal things about myself on the television and became convinced that I was being observed by CCTV in my room. The night before my final exams I went upstairs with a knife to prise open the floorboards and remove the cameras. The tenant upstairs was not about to let me in so I started forcing the door, and eventually he opened it.

As soon as I saw that inside there was a little, thin old man I knew that I was wrong. In the meantime he ran out of the room shrieking, and I was returning to my room to consider what to do next. As I was making my way downstairs another tenant to whom I had said hello a couple of times (and who had always blanked me in return) saw me with the knife, and although I have had many hallucinations I could swear that what he said next was not one of these. He said, 'Oh, another one has got out of his cell'. I just thought, 'fuck you mate', and I made for him and stabbed him in the side. Luckily it was only a flesh wound, and he ran downstairs to get help. I put the knife in my pocket and returned to my room to wait for the police.

When they arrived I gave them the knife and they handcuffed me, although I was not cautioned. I remember thinking 'how am I going to redeem this situation', and the words of a PhD student in the bar of the LSE came to mind. He had said, 'before you can become a doctor you must have a great fall, in order that you may rise again'. Although I understand now what he meant, at the time I was thinking that if only I could throw myself out of the window then I could rise again like the Phoenix. The policeman commented on how hot it was in the room and I tried to convince him to open the window. He took me out of the room, however, and delivered me to Kensington police station. At this stage I was in a state of shock and they called a doctor who gave me some Temazepam to help me sleep. The following day the police, observing the state that I was still in, called in an 'appropriate adult' before interviewing me. I gave a 'no comment' interview and was charged with GBH, which with hindsight was a bit excessive as the injuries were not grievous (here I must commend the police for their professionalism throughout). I went to court and I was remanded to

HMP Brixton.

When I arrived there I was, for the first time, suicidal, as I felt that those who were conspiring against me had finally succeeded. I was missing my exams. I was charged with a serious criminal offence. I felt that my mission had been scuppered. I felt that the only thing left for them to do was to take my life in order to cover up their conspiracy, and so I thought and believed that the other prisoners were planning to drown me in the hospital wing where I was staying. There was also a scaffold erected in the main entrance and I thought that there might also be a hanging. I felt that I had to resign myself to this fate.

After about a week in the hospital wing I was brought to see the doctor, then another doctor a few hours later, and the next thing I knew I was in a taxi on my way to Horton Secure Mental Hospital, where I was diagnosed as a paranoid schizophrenic. They asked me whether I was prepared to take medication and I said that I would be. I felt that I had nothing left to lose, although I did fear that they were going to try to brainwash me into being an Englishman. I took the first oral medication that they gave me, but nobody had warned me of the terrible side effects so I decided that I would not take any more. I was unable to control my face and my tongue was in and out of my mouth so much that I thought I was going to choke. For about six hours nurses and psychiatrists passed me by without bothering to explain that not all medication would have the same side-effects. I was completely in their power under a section 37, and they did not feel the need to seek my consent in anything that they wanted to do to me.

I remember in one group therapy session the therapist said, 'is there anything anyone wants to talk about?' and I said at the top of my voice 'Yes, RAPE'! They just ignored me and carried on.

I was still having auditory and visual hallucinations as I was not now taking the medication. Although we were supervised, I managed to spit it out for about three months. During this period I was constantly on the 'phone to solicitors, not realising just how powerful mental health sections are. I was asking them to seek injunctions against my treatment and to have it stopped, because I was afraid I was going to be injected and the symptoms I had encountered on my previous experience with medication would return and last for weeks, or until I choked to death.

After about three months they decided to start injecting me, and for two days I walked around with a biro intending to stab anyone who came near me with a needle. Eventually about a dozen of them surrounded me and told me that I was having the injection either with or without my consent. As they came closer I realised that I couldn't stab just one of them, and I consented to the injection. Fortunately the side effects were minimal this time, and so I agreed to further injections. After about three weeks the hallucinations had stopped completely, and, with them, my belief in a conspiracy. I was advised by my solicitor to plead 'not guilty but insane' to the charge, but I was afraid that if I did then I might end up not having a criminal record but being sent to Broadmoor or Rampton: so when I went to court I told my barrister that I would plead guilty to the lesser charge of malicious wounding. I did this and was remanded back to Horton, and after about a week I was transferred to the Chelsea and Westminster hospital as that was the area where I lived.

It was while I was there that the LSE awarded me an agreotat degree. This meant little to me at the time because I really felt that I had failed, not only at the LSE but in my mission to bring about a united Ireland. I didn't accept the agreotat degree, but I didn't refuse it either.

I was discharged from the Chelsea and Westminster after a couple of months, without a CPA (Community Psychiatric Assessment) meeting, and put into a B&B in Earl's Court. I was completely suicidal and my sister had me admitted again within 24 hours. After a while I was discharged again, this time into 91 Tavistock Street, a mental health hostel. I was very depressed and suicidal at this time. I was on Prozac, 50ml of intravenous Modecate once a fortnight and Procyclidine, an anti side-effect drug for the Modecate. I basically felt that my life was over bar the funeral, and all it consisted of was sleeping to 12:30 in the day, getting up for lunch, watching 'Home & Away', going back to bed at 3:30pm and sleeping until six. Then I would get up for dinner and watch television until 9:30, before returning to my bed and sleeping until 12:30 the next day.

For all of this period I was unable to communicate in a conversation. I could answer a direct question, but that was about the extent of it. The only change to my routine came on Fridays when I would cook shepherd's pie for the whole of the hostel. This went down well at first, but they were all really sick to the back teeth of it after a year. At about this time I began actually considering suicide. I had a good drink and I when up to the top of the high-rise in Euston where I had used to live, but I could not jump. I then walked down to the Thames and thought for an hour about jumping in, but I became convinced that I would probably be pulled out so I abandoned that idea. Eventually, after many deliberations, I decided on an overdose.

One night I went to bed earlier than usual and took 72 Prozac: as they were anti-depressants, I thought that they would do the job, but I only awoke again to a great disappointment and feeling very drowsy. I had basically slept for about three days, but as I was sleeping so much anyway it all went unnoticed.

The only changes over the next two years were that of my Irish stew period, which lasted for about a year, and my lasagne period, which also lasted around twelve months.

After I had been in the hostel for about three years I decided to reduce my medication. Instead of going every two weeks for my depot injection I went once every three, effectively reducing my intake by 50%. Through this I felt able to do a night class in Spanish. Although still reticent, I was able to communicate slightly better.

After fifteen months of defaulting on the drug, I got the first ever appointment with my Consultant Psychiatrist. When he asked me how I was I told him, 'I am not the person I used to be'; whereas I had used to talk, argue, and generally hold my own in any conversation I was now very taciturn, unable to communicate and quiet. He told me that my medication, as well as having anti-psychotic effects was also a sedative, and that we should consider reducing my intake further. We decided on cutting it down to 50ml every month, and on stopping the Procyclidine completely, unless needed.

The change that this brought about was quite dramatic: within about three weeks I was out chatting up girls again, talking about religion, politics, sex, anything. I felt I had five years of talking still inside of me. I also enrolled on a course, 'giving advice on benefits & welfare rights'.

I decided that I wanted to train as a Citizens' Advice Bureaux volunteer, and then after maybe five years return to pursue politics in the Republic of Ireland.

I claimed my agreotat degree from the LSE and you know what they say about agreotat degrees, they could be a pass or they could be a first. Personally, I consider mine to be a first.

AN UPHILL STRUGGLE, BUT IT'S BEEN WORTH IT

FRANK BANGAY

I don't see myself as a victim. Survivors of mental health services experience some horrifying things; we need to talk about them, and society needs to hear some of the real horror stories, but the public shouldn't see us as victims.

The general public wouldn't normally read a book about mental health and we're often treated with suspicion, but we need to be able to get our messages across, to show what we can achieve with our creativity and campaigns, and also what it's like to go through these often horrific experiences and what it's like to be discriminated against.

You can't change the whole of society with a poem, but if you can help someone to understand things a little more and they go away and think and talk to a friend, you start to help change attitudes and break barriers down. The mental health survivor groups I've been involved in, of which one member, Eric Irwin, was a very strong speaker, have done workshops in front of mental health professionals. While they have had an impact, we usually encountered the doubting thomases who wanted to contradict what we were saying. But then sometimes I've read a poem and it has helped to drive a point home.

For me, poetry has always been a lifeline, and about having a fighting spirit, whether the issues being touched on are personal or political. It's not always easy to get poetry across to an audience. People get touchy about certain subjects, and if you're talking about psychiatry, at some venues you might possibly be told to shut up. But there are important things that we need to say, and we need to confront stereotypes and show that we're not dangerous people.

Survivor poets have always been around. It could be argued that in England they go back at least to people like John Clare and William Blake. There were survivor poets who I met in the late 1970s and 1980s: one who left an impression on me was a chap called Rod Stuart. I met him in 1973; however, he had been writing poetry long before that. He was a well-travelled and experienced person, and a number of his poems addressed survivor issues. His poetry was rooted deeply in life experience, and he gave hope to many, even during difficult times. He died in 1981, and people who knew him saw his death as a tragedy, and will always remember his poetry. I still have copies of some of his poems.

The organisation *Survivors' Poetry* followed directly from a history of struggle by survivors of the mental health system. Out of the Mental Patients Union grew PROMPT (Promotion of the Rights of Mental Patients in Treatment), which itself evolved into CAPO - the Campaign Against Psychiatric Oppression. These weren't poetry groups, they were campaigning groups, but poetry has always been an important part of the struggle. Part of the idea for *Survivors' Poetry* came from CAPO benefit gigs, the PROMPT publication *Mixed Emotions* and the CAPO publications *What They Teach In Song* and *Rhythm of Struggle, Song of Hope*, which included both articles and poetry in order to combine our ideology and personal experience.

During the late 1970s and early 1980s I knew a lot of survivor poets who died due to their life struggles, and this inspired me to fight for acceptance for our collective voice. However, *Survivors' Poetry* brought together a variety of influences. When it got going in the early 90s, a large number of poets and folk musicians who'd used mental health services were becoming visible on the London performance circuit - people like Pauline Bradley, Anna Neeter and Peter Campbell, as well as performers like Sam Green and Dave Russell who had been around for many years. Suddenly there were enough of us around, and it was the right time to make it happen.

Traditionally, poets struggle to get spots to read poems about mental health issues. When poets tried to do it at venues like the Troubadour, there was the risk that someone might start heckling, or accusing the poet of being paranoid for speaking out about such things. This was an experience I often had, and it could designate you a stereotyped role, though the CAPO benefits there helped to change this a bit. We'd all had a lot of experience of rejection, and we wanted to try to make our own space, for ourselves, to perform and to learn.

Joe Bidder, Hilary Porter and Bushy Kelly, who worked for the Arts Council and organised the initial funding, came along with their own different life experiences and organisational skills, and *Survivors' Poetry* was born, the first gig being in Autumn 1991 at the Toriano Meeting House in Kentish Town, run by the anarchist poet John Retty. We did two performances there before moving to the Hampden Community Centre, now known as Somerstown Community Centre, where monthly shows still take place.

I have fond memories of the heyday of *Survivors' Poetry*, during the first half of the 1990s. It gave many people a chance to develop their confidence and perform, providing them with a platform when there was nowhere else. I organised and co-organised many events in day centres, sheltered housing and other psychiatric settings. Some of these events were very positive and I enjoyed this work immensely. There was a time when I lived in a mental health hostel and the staff were trying to push the work ethic, making everyone go out every day and look for a job. If a group like *Survivors' Poetry* had come into the hostel then and done a workshop or a gig, I'd have had the chance to read poems and get involved and it would have helped me and maybe other residents a lot. It may also have helped the staff there understand a little about the value of creativity.

I've always believed that survivors of the mental health system can have a confident voice, and that survivor poets have the right to perform alongside other types of radical poetry. However, when *Survivors' Poetry* tried to encompass a wider network of interests, many of the original ideas were lost.

The definition of 'survivor' began to widen and people who hadn't used psychiatric services started to get involved, and I felt that the voice of psychiatric system survivors was marginalised. People with more socially acceptable and therefore more powerful voices began to get the lion's share of attention, and it led to a struggle within the group. The aim of *Survivors' Poetry* originally was to help people gain confidence and get taken seriously, but for radical mental health survivors, this aim became more distant. It felt sometimes that we were battling to make ourselves heard above people who began to seem condemning, even prejudiced.

Restrictions by funders were partly at the root of this. As *Survivors' Poetry* expanded, it increasingly became answerable to funders, and Arts Council funded poets who weren't in the strictest sense survivors had to be booked to keep them happy. While I think it's fine if people want to learn by performing with us, the fact is that sometimes they might do so only to improve their CVs. It often went wrong and there were poets who wouldn't get a favourable response from a grass roots audience.

Things became more restrictive. I became less involved, and felt like an outsider in the work that I was trying to do and in my views. I felt that *Survivors' Poetry* had gone off track. Funders like the arts council shouldn't be necessary for survivor poets, because they favour professional poets who can't afford to be too rebellious. This encourages grass roots poets, and activities like workshops in sheltered housing, to be overlooked. It also makes the aims of *Survivors' Poetry* more wide-ranging and therefore more vague. There are a lot of causes outside of mental health that need to be talked about, and there are many different kinds of oppressive regimes, but they are often linked to psychiatry, and issues of psychiatry and surviving the system can get left out if they're not given space. Even the selection processes involved in the *Survivors' Poetry* anthologies began to reflect these tensions.

A group like CAPO would have looked at oppressive regimes elsewhere, but it would also have looked directly at the links with what was happening in our own field. As mental health survivors, we have our own experience and history of campaigning and creating alternatives going back at least to the early 1970s, which need to be acknowledged separately, not just as part of the wider disability world. I like and respect many of the poets associated with it and have befriended some people in the disability movement, and many survivors have disabilities, but it already has more of a means to make its interests heard. While it is important to link up and campaign about issues which affect us all, such as benefits cuts, we need to hang onto our own history and acknowledge our own struggle for rights. Otherwise, our views are diluted.

This said, there have been very many things I've loved about *Survivors' Poetry*. In particular, the new survivor poets who developed their acts through workshops and had the chance to perform at the Hampden Community Centre, and the good receptions I've had there for my own performances. The concerns I've expressed about the direction *Survivors' Poetry* was taking are a reflection of the group as it was while I was still involved; they are not meant as an attack on the current group. I'll never forget the times when many of us shared common aims and seemed to know where each other were coming from. And of course, there will always be the writing, the poems.

TOWARDS A CRITICAL MADNESS
BEN WATSON

The box-file with the legend "OTL: MADOBILIA 1983" on its spine is raspberry pink, exactly the same pink as a single ceramic boot with a yellow lace I bought in a Horsforth giftshop during the lunch-hour in 1984. The same pink as Esther's desk in fact (my, weren't the 80s a vicious, pink decade!). The colour is mouthwatering in a synthetic kind of way. The thing looks smooth and slick, like a rhubarb-fool flavour penny-chew. There's something threatening about it, like a vinyl fetish sex-toy glimpsed by chance on an operating table in a rundown hospital in North Wales. If you licked the shiny surface, it would clog the pores of your tongue: an over-inquisitive housefly drowning in a tin of pink emulsion.

But I don't lick the box. I sit with it in my lap. I'm writing these words on the first page of a lined file-pad balanced on top of the box. I'll draw it for you. I place a blank piece of drawing paper on top of the file-pad. Blank paper on lined paper on raspberry pink; all on my lap.

I can see a plaster on my right heel, a blister sustained dancing to Alternative TV at their Mad Pride gig at the Union Chapel, Highbury & Islington. Or was it the Sex Machine covers band later on at the Hen & Chicken? Or the walk home to Somers Town, limping behind Esther and Josh, a mysterious pair loitering at street corners in a deadquiet nightblack Islington? Another London punkrock motif is my Diary t-shirt with the anti-NATO/pro-Serb target symbol. I think I'll move this pad I'm writing on (transcribing from, now, RSI juddering down the sinews of my wrist, alleviated by a can of Grolsch). Now my writing pad is resting on the arm of the chair. I'm looking at the exposed surface of the box-file. I can see my head outlined against the reflection of the window behind me. Unevenness in the surface wobbles the light.

Before I even open the box and stir these reminders of my lunatic past, the way my head floats over the surface - eyeless, misshapen, sinister flat-top, ears dissolving into panes of light - makes me anxious. Any Marxist who'd want to explore psychoanalysis needs their head examined.

Here I am then. I'm examining my head, and, mum, I'm scared! There is nothing more surreal than sitting in an armchair and making concrete observations. Who needs TV! This is our alternative! (Perry Marks the spot in pearshaped bubbles.) I open the box (suppressing the impulse to use the "poetic" "ope'").

On top of a thick wedge of assorted scrap paper - madpersons'll write on anything, you know - there's a copy of *Materialism and Empirio-Criticism* by Vladimir Lenin, cream-coloured Chinese Communist softback edition from the late 70s, when such rare morsels could be had for 10p. The cover's revolutionary severity has been tampered with, though. There's a glued-on picture of a spooky old house, steep roofs and narrow workhouse windows. It's been cut from a postcard and stuck over another cutting, a postcard photo of an artificial lake - note the straight edge of the dam - in a verdant valley. Also, a murky brown cutting of three cows crossing a ford (Constable?) by the edge of the lake. A humorous montagiste without much care for perspective or realism, I surmise. Up above, something completely at variance to this idyll: a wedge-shaped cutting with a print of small spherical objects in different colours - white, orange, green. Eerie hints of psychiatric medication? Hallucinatory drugs? Hallucinatory drugs liberated from a psychiatric institution, perhaps? An addiction to x-rays leading to fraudulent hospitalization? It's been cut in a shape that suggests an aeroplane crash-landing on the house. Maybe a missile primed with mind-deranging chemicals? Agent Ridgeway Kool-Aid Orange laced with LSD? A monster vision in the placid lake? Tired of the questionmarks required at the end of each of these phrases, I open up the book.

Someone's been let loose on the title page, mad graffiti abounds. 'WORKERS OF ALL LANDS, UNOTE!' it says, a blue hand-driven felt tip interfering with Maoist red-type correctness. Unote: you note, take note, one note ... union-chapel toke? And in this cup an onion shall I throw! Unote, united note, one note ... the Big Note, the cosmic monochord beloved of Pythagorian mystics. The original owner's name has been

scratched out. Instead she's written in my own name and the date.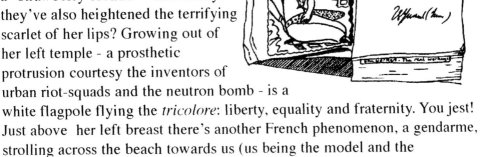
Boning the owner in a rain of kittens, it's 29/10/83! (How nineteenth-
century and past-it these dates look as we cross year 2000). Uncanny to see
one's own name written in another's hand. Loopy girly script, blue biro - a
writing implement I'd never use.

Overleaf, a kitsch postcard of a dolly-bird on the beach. Tipped-in by the
mad montagiste. The beauty is wearing an itsy-bitsy polka-dot bikini and a
gold bracelet; a gold ring on one
finger, nail varnish, dark blue shoe
with a strap. There's a sun-umbrella
up above, tassels. Her hair's been
coloured-in by the postcard makers,
an amazing burnished copper colour -
a "strawberry blonde" - and surely
they've also heightened the terrifying
scarlet of her lips? Growing out of
her left temple - a prosthetic
protrusion courtesy the inventors of
urban riot-squads and the neutron bomb - is a
white flagpole flying the *tricolore*: liberty, equality and fraternity. You jest!
Just above her left breast there's another French phenomenon, a gendarme,
strolling across the beach towards us (us being the model and the
photographer), his serge-blue form materializing from the out-of-focus
middle-distance.

On the recto, it's the classic Maoist "photograph" of Lenin, his face
shining after the Stalinist air-brush. His lips appear to have been
contaminated by the kitsch postcard opposite (their lips are positioned to rest
together when you close the book). Lenin's lips have blushed a deep, dark
scarlet (reminiscent of the indelible dye O applies to her nipples and sex in
Return To The Château). His impudent rictus grimaces at the onlooker, a
camp little pout. His collar has been coloured-in with a pink highlighter. It
looks like it's blushing with shame. Sex in the house of Communism! WR:
Mysteries Of The Organism restaged inside the covers of a book! Folded in
four inside the volume - a bookmark perhaps? - is a leaflet headed
'NALGO's Day Of Inaction', issued by the Communist Workers
Organisation of Glasgow. I take it out and peruse the text, appreciating the
old-world stencil-and-roneo greyness and typos. After the leaflet's
predictable denunciation of everybody and everything, there's a note in
hand-written biro:

"See above for the best politics in the world. The ultra-left musical
tosspot can't be kept down. Come round 'n hear my favourite 12"

disco single."

Irony from a bolshevik ice maiden? It's like Chris Knight asking Stewart Home, "Do you hold nothing sacred?" Home: "I'm a materialist - I don't deal with religious concepts." Knight: "I'm a revolutionary communist but I can't see where you're coming from." Home: "Them over there, they're in the SWP, and they're not offended!" Chris Knight: "What's the SWP line on blow jobs?" What a question to hear in Camden High Street Waterstone's! It all depends on the individual member, Chris. Political seriousness dissolves in a welter of *Carry On*-style innuendo (what're you reading a book on Mad Pride for if you want to be *serious*?) "That old mole our mock-seriousness digs deeper than your perimeter fencing, sad victim of anthropo-mystical mind-boggling, we enclude the material universe and every thought therein, great and small, serious and obscene, holy and profane ..." The Mad Dietzgenite mutter beneath the sober prose.

Back to the book in hand. It's evident that the molester of this piece of Maoist propaganda, Agent Ridgeway, is a plant, determined to locate my sex diaries and use my endless desire for loose sexual dalliance as a means of detumescing the rigour of my Leninist critique. Neon-pink flashes of orgone energy, sharp scent of burning zinc. Paradoxically, the call to revolutionary discipline is arousing me as well, the fear manufacturing hormones in waves. That reference to her 12" ... is she actually a transvestite or just a hermaphrodite? Or is she taking the piss, punishing me for fecklessness and irresponsibility? Fear, guilt and arousal pursue each other across my emotional template like the three-legged swastika cut into the plateglass window of the Three Legs pub on Leeds Headrow. I unstick one side of the crimped kitsch postcard and peer beneath (blushing slightly at my unseemly curiosity): "Happy Birthday," I read, "Best wishes for a successful Revolution" ...

Head and cock throbbing from this sex attack - the peculiar way those spiked with madness can actually *smell* sex-arousal chemicals emanating from those on-heat foxes, slathering mastiffs & eager bitches - I rifle through the pages, determined to find more clues to the enigma of Agent Ridgeway. Her name swims before my eyes ... ridge ... way ... hiking across a mountain ridge, the opposite of a chasm, a kind of negative abyss, the opposite of cunt, a *tnuc* - "TN, you see?" TN? Too Naff!! In the back, mad graffiti of my own devise: "Danny may last for the durex ... But I've got my finger on the triggah"; "Steve Gaunt was FZ and JCF Hall!"; "Bit of everyday thing in EVERYTHING."

The myth of individuality is an illusion produced by bourgeois property relations - the attempt to press the potential of mass-production into inheritance patterns that imitate the bloodlines of the aristocrats. No human mind can truly cognise more than five other human psyches in the world; our unconscious is no more advanced than the hunter-gatherer grouplet. That's why genocide and third-world starvation persist despite the advances of technology. All past civilisations have foundered on this simple error, as ruling classes take decisions whose real impact on people's lives - felt from inside, subjectively, humanly - they can't feel, imagine or conceptualize. Though you use ledgers and diaries and calendars and address books to try and differentiate the "actual" people who've passed through your life, you cannot really cope with life's stream of characters and types and names. You reduce everyone to your restricted set of personal archetypes. The softspoken boy in glasses in 2B who you quite liked merges with Tom in 6C who behaved the same. All doctors will always be Doctor Mike to you (or "Ekim," as he signed his first Christmas card to you). You only ever fall in love with Jane Thomas, the tomboy with the red-golden curls who lived nextdoor to your cousin on High Park Road across the railway track. You only ever admire the intellect of someone who reminds you of Jerry - who showed you how to make liquorice water and write four-letter words down in scurrilous books (burning excitement of Thoth, the mystic shaman, your guide to mucking with semantics). There's only ever been one boss you've hated. These truths are humiliating to admit to, puncture the ambition of the great historical manipulators and politicians, reduce politics to honesty among a small group of peers - a central committee, a revolutionary cell. The idea of an instant communication between a leading genius and millions of people is a fascist/communist fantasy. Today's version is perpetrated by Rupert Murdoch and Bill Gates.

A packet of 35mm film. The envelope has been scribbled on with black felt-tip: "Ben bonkers" and "Cumbernauld Road, Glasgow." The images are hard to make out, pale colour negatives. I recognise some of them. They were taken after I'd discovered that Poundstretcher on Vicar Lane was selling George Clinton's *One Nation Under A Groove* - shrinkwrapped, *with* the 33rpm single "Lunchmeataphobia (Think! It Ain't Illegal Yet!)" (essential possession for a punk called Out To Lunch) - for 10p a throw. I spent £2 of my giro and a year giving them away to friends (Dr Mike ended up with two, I recall). Walked across Leeds city centre with an armful of Clinton vinyl, smile on my face. Then I arranged them all around the room, a frieze of pink-and-green eye-candy to zap the iris. Pedro Bell cracked the Mayan mystic secret which Charles Olson yearned to find; the ability to improvise coloured symbols that wreak and accentuate twists on the neurones of the brain. It packs an intensity that bourgeois realism - with its monotonous single-point perspective (everything rushing down the tunnel of death) and boring deep brown shadows - can never lock into.

Rearrange objects in the house! That was the first abacus, the proto-computer. Turn over a book that's lying at the top of the stairs and the whole equation shifts. The house is but an external symbol of the thinking mind (how Esther can work in her lumber room of tottering bookpiles is beyond me). Just as a single new concept can provide the slogan for an entire period of social transformation, so a rearranged room in a single house configures an entire new epoch. That's what Kurt Schwitters understood when he built his various *Merzbauen*. Bugger the gallery and the art sales and the applauded limelight of the curated mausoleum, it's the thought that counts! My frieze of Funkadelic albums was a plagiarist one-man show, a Neoist exhibition so underground no-one ever heard of it (until now, and all you readers are insane and mad, so what the fuck!?).

Exhibitionist multiples expose the mass-productive capacity behind the existence of commercially-available records, a fact kept hidden by careful price structuring and warehouse storage - impounding social property in order to force up the price. The record industry: the most heinous charade of the entire capitalist racket! We're encouraged to think we're individuals, living our determinate and specific and private lives, but we're all in the same gaol: watching the same TV, cracking the same "new" jokes, commenting on the same massaged scrap of news, eating the same fake food, farting the same (real) farts. Out To Lunch's Funkadelikus-in-Maximalia eye-popper - Splankalicious! - boiled down this pseudo-individualism to its mass base. Multiplistic duplication pointed to duplication everywhere. This exhibit marked the birth of post-postmodern Mass Man, de-evolved, free to embrace the radical de-individualised post-property equality of mass-produced wealth. A subversive *denouement*, an installation that exaggerated and redoubled the capitalist order until the system would feedback, override and crash.

Madness is just Modern Art without the authoritarian intimidation - the essays that make you wanna puke, the lectures that make you wanna kill someone, the auction values that line some dealer's pocket, the catalogue that makes some bureaucrat's career - to force respect from minds that cannot inkle its utopian promises. Why bother with the rigmarole? Anyone intimidated into recognising Modern Art will never sense its secret - the intimation of a world without fear.

There is a difference, though, between Madness and Art that's not entirely on Madness's side. Now I'm no longer screaming heebie-jeebies mad and no longer entertaining alternate visions/theories/scenarios every hour - expecting the flying saucers and the revolution and the apocalypse and the Nazis and the last judgement in permutative succession - what's re-turned is my ability to live in the present order, to manipulate social status. Or

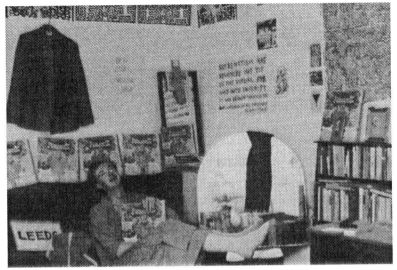

res-
tored
my collusion
with it, my
insensitivity
to its crimes?
It's still a
quandary.
The joy of
madness is
the evap-
oration of the
insignificance
capitalism
condemns us to. That's why it's like art.

Ever since the age of sixteen I've made cut-ups of whatever's in my waste-
paper basket (Freud called his *Interpretation Of Dreams* "my own dung
heap"). Not random cut-ups as publicised by William Burroughs and Brion
Gysin, but *Merz* ... I'll have to explain. The Madness started after seeing an
exhibition by Kurt Schwitters in the Marlborough Gallery on Old Bond
Street (I'd learned that if you have the "front" you can walk in these places
and look about, see some brand new art for free). I was completely thrilled
that someone could take old bus tickets and sweet wrappers and toothless
combs and worn-out brooms with flaking paint and rusty pram wheels and -
just by being electrically sensitive to colour and shape and joky nuance -
craft something that seemed to shine off the gallery walls, hovering patches
of Modern Art that were more effective and bewitching and glorious than
anything by Picasso or Kandinsky, or even Mondrian. Co-ordinated rubbish
could be more beautiful than any icon made of gold and pearls, more real and
urban and modern than any oil-painting, however advanced its way of
seeing! You stared-in close at a Schwitters' Merz (he had to invent a word for
what he did, "collage" sounds like something made of coloured tissue paper
or cuttings from colour supplements; a "montage" implies clean, hard-
focused photographs ... Schwitters' materials all reek!), and every one is full
of mad puns and references and mindbending absurdities, chock-a-block with
real information about everyday life in Berlin and Hanover in the 20s and
30s - but also insane and colourful and poetic. Like life actually is. No boring
"once upon a time', no tedious *mis-en-scène*, no chiarascuro or tender
evocation requiring plot and lighting and stage-management - but bits of past
time's *actualities* stuck all over the picture surface! Schwitters' Merz
collations wriggle and burn with infantile charm and subversion. A

Modern Art anything-goes Rabelais, a visual *Finnegans Wake*, a tramp-who-would-be-king, another member of the true secret humble vainglorious *literati* to engage in jest with! Kurt Schwitters, the best thing to hit the twentieth century. For, Comrades ... Rubbish Is Pertinent!

But why am I telling you this? Because, although I'm proud to have gone Mad, and I treasure the Madness that I know still lurks beneath the brim of my being, I don't like the collages and drawings and poems I made when I was Mad ...

I would hallucinate and try and draw the vision floating on the page. Dragons, milkmaids, wooded valleys. The images always came out limp, without the tension and aboriginal twang of insectoid-and-hieratic-deco doodles, even. I'd use things for their symbolic value rather than the way they looked, scraping a curly banana across the page to express lust, rubbing capers into a letter-head to show I was capable of anything. Too much white paper, too much scribble, too little craft. Too much use of matches - scorch marks on everything. I even put a match to my favourite bluegrass record, Reno and Smiley's *Greatest Hits* on Gusto (was it because Helen said they looked like members of the Ku Klux Klan? - vile rubbish thing to say). My Mad Merz period looks like magic remnants - used, burnt, sordid - nothing inspiring, no food for the eye. I'd use materials that wouldn't last, like orange peel. Mad Pride is about being proud of what we discover by going mad, not overvaluing every scrap and issue of total social dislocation. Maybe that's why only Normals can be fans of Antonin Artaud - they haven't seen the puke on the lino in a nut-house, experienced the chill of imagining life as that grey and institutional and miserable forever. Why Artaud's "art" makes me cringe - it's the residue of psychosis curated by the comfortable rather than psychic weaponry to arm the proletariat. (Yes, Rob wrote the introduction, not me.)

Madness showed me something true - a life lived in the instant, for the instant, respecting and playing with the people right there in the room as if they were the whole universe - but I'll have to drag the rest of society round to my point of view to prove it. If there wasn't any pressure to accumulate capital and everyone was provisioned and housed - a minor task for today's productive capability - then history would open up into infinity: each life could became an end in itself instead of a drab statistic. If everyone was inventing themselves on the basis of provision and no fear, then every household and street you encounter would be a total trip, another universe. But to try and live like that here and now risks destitution, begging, violence, incarceration. To still hold onto what my Madness meant, I have to address the consciousness bred by capitalism - privatised, possessive, competitive, driven by fear of homelessness and ruin, scared by the future right unto death.

At moments, though, we *can* unfurl the red banner and get a glimpse - bizarre flashes - of our Mad Utopia: the selfless collective wager made by strikers, the solidarity of anti-fascist mobilisations, the invention and adventure of the riot. Did you notice how the Nude Protest people could walk about at the June 18th Carnival Against Capitalism totally unmolested, laughed with, celebrated? What kind of psychosis is everyone else living that public nudity must mean outrage, violence, oppression, horror? In 1917 they staged a naked demonstration in Leningrad - "Against Shame!"

For me, time spent on a Merz construction is a moment of resistance to the way colour and shape is exploited by the commodity system (most of my sources are packaging; after all, this is what lies about us all the time ...). To do this stuff so it doesn't replicate the patterns I object to requires ingenuity and care. Fuck "being an artist" and flogging the things! The ABC of authentic resistance. These are the issues Simon and Rob must consider every time they organise a Mad Pride event. It was the central concern of original punk. Machines for making money are tedious and expensive charades; the punter stupidity hangs in the air like a foul miasma. If the economic transaction is exploitative, the event can only be a carnival of false consciousness. That's why the best gigs are around politics - or entered by breaking in at the back - or stumbled on by accident. It was seeing Killing Joke and Spear Of Destiny in quick succession - hack rock bands, jumping punters, smiling promoters, no aggro, no event - that made me abandon punk for Free Improvisation and Jazz. Find me a musical form that'll never make the bossmen any money! I could never understand why John Peel always kept his ears at the 15-years-old level. Of course "art" has its own sicknesses and boredoms and career-structure too. What would Ornette Coleman make of Mark Perry's violin playing? Why don't these people talk to each other? Separation, the imprint of the Iron Heel.

Madness has always fringed revolutionary politics and the art scene because both are predicated on transgression of oppressive social norms. It's the craft and discipline of Marxism and of Modern Art to allow in a certain amount of strategy and calculation without losing the point. The anarchy symbol at the heart of Mad Pride is probably the only one that'll do - with its intimations of POUM and punk and stop-the-city riots - but anarchism's hatred of reflection and theory causes endless paradox, suspicion and treachery. There's no rational yardstick in this area! The Mad dropping away of socialised conscience (*aka* Freud's superego) can simply reveal solipsism, megalomania, star-struck fantasies - enough anti-social psychosis to confirm the repressions of every bourgeois liberal. That is why we need a Critical Madness, a madness driven by revolutionary consciousness, though not necessarily bound into party structures or tenets. After all, it's because Madness strips away the super-ego - and that includes political ideology, social conscience, sense of history and political correctness - that it makes the actuality of the treatment of human beings here and now the absolute terrain of discussion. Only those without property, power or special interests can contribute to this process.

Too much bloody preaching, baby. I thought this was Mad Pride! Let's see what's in the box ...

A section of wallpaper torn from the stairwell, 29 Glossop Street, Woodhouse, Leeds 6. Written in loopy green wax-crayon, you can make out the words "do it ... ugh, JT." It's a message for Johnny Thunders, a reference to his song "It's Not Enough" on *L.A.M.F.* I was obsessed with Johnny Thunders (I still am - the only American "punk" worth caring about, the only one with that jesuitical streak injected the wrong way, the only Italian whiteboy-with-soul who ever walked the streets of NYC, the only inheritor of the funky-ruff mantle of Jerry Lee Lewis, the plangent cross-tied bleeding-heart of any debate about the heart of a heartless world - how could you let us down and die, Johnny? I exit weeping ...).

I went to see Johnny Thunders sometime between Christmas and New Year, 1983, Camden Dingwalls. I met up with Agent Ridgeway there. We snogged over the chrome railing at the front, we drank bottles of beer. It was fantastic! There was some broken glass near the entrance, almost like a little installation to instil punk fear among the punters, a challenge to see who'd use it in a fight. Or just a bottle someone broke. Who knows? In my delusion, I believed that "Johnny Thunders" was just the temporary name for any totally deadbeat wreck with spindly legs and a leather jacket and mascara who the promoters could get on stage to strum a guitar. Like "Sun Ra" is just the folkloric moniker for any blubbery middle-aged old fraud who can blow iridescent bubbles and tell us stories from his bathtub, amaze the children staring through the keyholes - kaleidoscopes, fairy-lights, absurdly cheap synthesizers, news of outer space: Sostenuto, *we're off to Pluto*, wow!

There was a long delay at Dingwalls. We all stood around drinking and waiting. No support band as I recall. The promoters were scouring the pubs of Camden looking for a "Johnny Thunders." Anyone would do. It's like finding a Pearly King or a Carnival Queen. Maybe they'd pick me! They eventually found a geezer, requisite spindly legs in black jeans, shock of black hair. Was it Thunders or John Cooper Clarke (now, he turned up on June 18th ...)? He sang a set of three Bob Dylan songs, Lou Reed's "Vicious", and then fell over. So un-punk and funny ... me and Agent Ridgeway snogged some more. I hope Esther doesn't object to these reminiscences. You can only reminisce about love affairs that are well and truly over, you know. The ongoing thing, well, mind your own business.

Mark Perry sounds just like Thunders on the tracks produced by Steve Albini on Alternative TV's *Punk Life*. Songs from the whining broken-down boy with nothing to his name, the true lyricism of the proletariat. "It's not enough ..." whinges Johnny; "DO IT ENOUGH!" quoth Lunch, one eye on Wilhelm Reich's *The Sexual Revolution*, another on Johnny's junkie fingers nicking a few more rare-as-hen's-teeth singles on the Dot label to punt for his habit.

Writing on the walls - the practice of children, mad persons and old-skool hip-hop gang-bangers. Those who run the real rackets write their names in neon or plastic or brass: Tescos, McDonalds, the British Museum. But let me explain about the significance of the stairwell for Out To Lunch on a Madness trip. It's predicated on a theory, of course.

What everyone wants, tortured by the tedium of capitalism-as-usual, is a P-A-R-T-Y (and I don't mean a political organisation, chuck). But the *real* party-out-of-bounds is a dangerous thing, man, a B52 bomber, a fucker to let off! There is an ineluctable drive to wreck the private living space, because privacy and decorum baulks the idea that everyday life could be a continuous PARTY. What's it like, the party-out-of-bounds, then? Searing smell of burnt zinc, the house suddenly invaded by mysteriously attractive, slyly smiling people with bottles under their arms and make-up on their faces. Weird new people dancing strange new dances (like The Uranium-Depleted), plus old friends I haven't seen for years looking incongruously - but shiningly - young. Everyone's wearing ludicrous parody-suits and jumble-sale dresses, Gerry slips a Frankenstein's monster rubber-mask over my head. It's clammy, but the movement of bodies is, well, exciting. They're pouring 70° absinthe from a slim green bottle, flaming the sugar over my kitchen table, someone's making great gloopy oversize soap bubbles at the sink, they're outing my Iggy Pop and Johnny "Guitar" Watson albums. There are party hats and crackers and streamers and poppers. People wearing clownsuits tapping at the windows, sound of laughter in the street. Wild. They've started drawing wild artistic hilarious obscene pictures all over the walls with expensive Caran d'Ache pastels, they're drawing them on the ceiling (a human pyramid which collapses in hysterical laughter), they're heading up the stairwell. The phone is ringing, they've set off both my alarm clocks, there are Techno tapes and sex tapes and parrot tapes running on every tape-machine in the house. The noise is horrendous, the party hysteria is mounting and mounting.

The crescendo is almost classical - am I dreaming this? - suddenly someone shouts "scramble!" and everyone's diving for the doors and windows, multiple sound of shattering glass. I've only just registered that the guests have all gone - there's a pierrot's slipper protruding from between the radiator and the window-sill - when there's a deafening roar like a Xenakis orchestral climax, too loud to hear, and blackness envelopes me ...

I awake. Smell of burn. Rain on my face. I open my eyes. The roof has been blown clean off! I check myself for injury. Tear off my clothes, now just a bundle of scorched rags. Check myself. No injuries, nothing bad. Just "do it ...ugh" written in scarlet lipstick on my chest. I groan and lie back on the cindery floorboards, letting the flecks of rain cool my heated frame. Up above, the stars are so bright it's like they're bulging in the firmament. The Milky Way a swathe of light. To lie naked in the rain, wrote Christopher Smart, is to worship God ...

Leafing through the notes, poems and torn scraps and staplings in the raspberry-pink "madobilia" box-file, I understand why they've been herded together here, under quarantine, isolated from my other papers. They explode with hopes and plans that simply "weren't realistic". The tone is embarrassing, too. Along with the jumps of logic and mad puns ("She's insane - she's in Sainsbury's," as Gamma puts it), which I still enjoy, there's a gushing optimism and jubilant hallooing about revolution and socialism that make me cringe. I can understand why people committed to revolutionary politics should have a horror of madness. By saying what we want - egalitarianism, lives of direct human interaction and contact, participation in history: an end, in short, to alienation - we put ourselves outside the pale of convincing and effective discourse. In politics, as in music, time is everything - *when* to say that it's time to burst the bonds of capitalism. People who say it's now now now become a stuck clock - correct twice every 24 hours. What's wrong with the exhortations incarcerated in the box is not their intent or even the way they're phrased, but the lack of worldly cynicism about how daft they sound in the current climate. As silly as the preacher in the street calling for everyone to shed their property and believe in Jesus.

Is revolution made by the "dispossessed," the people *without anything* or by the WORKERS - those who've seized the means of production? Is there a mismatch between Hegelian negation and the Realpolitik of class warfare? No! It was actually the *lack* of control over the means of

116

production - workers retreating to the land/being massacred in the civil war - that meant the Soviet Union couldn't stand up for the dispossessed of the world. Empirical historical investigation solves political riddles abstract ratiocination won't teach you. When workers seize a factory we're told it no longer "belongs" to anybody: it's been taken out of the era of commodity exchange and into socialism. Dispossession *is* the state of socialised property!

Of course, Normals suffer too when they leaf through an old diary or a pile of love letters. As the poet JH Prynne once observed, the archive is a harmful place, and you don't go digging around in there with impunity. If you've forgotten something it's for a reason. It's the unprotected nature of the statements in the pink box-file - no assessment of the opposition, no assessment of future readers - that hurts, rather than the Madness. This is stuff anyone - Mad or Normal - quietly covers up to go on living in the present.

One of the most bewildering aspects of going Mad on the NHS is being incarcerated alongside the other nutters. When I was sectioned to Highroyds Mental Hospital I was undergoing an extreme case of character-recognition condensation. Not necessarily to classical-Freudian family archetypes, either. A toothless old guy standing by the ward lockers, grey, wrinkled and unshaven, was immediately Steptoe from *Steptoe & Son*. The plump young loonie with frizzy hair who strummed guitar in a tiny blind room off the main hall was immediately Bob Dylan. But then, that's who he said he was, so I was no doubt biased. After two weeks of medication in the closed ward - and numerous earnest conversations with the nurses I sensed had authority in the place - I was considered safe enough for the open section. The serenity after the pressure-cooker bedlam of the closed ward was unbelievable. A rectilinear brick 1940s building, steel window-frames, brown lino floors. In the outlying garden, low brick walls topped with square white stone, rose trellises, little brick-paved patios with restful deckchairs. Vista of green fields down to the river Aire. A cold wind blew in at the open French windows, though late summer sunshine still tempted patients out to watch the sunset.

At the open ward things were calm enough for patients to do art therapy. We'd mucked around with crayons and paint back in bedlam, but everyone was too frantic and interactive and attention-seeking to actually draw or paint anything. It occurs to me as I write this that I actually love the resistance of genuine psychological observation to "objective" study: if I start wondering whether loonie bins are semiotic regeneration tanks (if art's so irrelevant to science and economics, how come it's the most relied-on form of psychiatric cure? isn't money and data actually made by humans in the first place?), I'm pulled up by remembering that art and writing are "my" things anyway. What I was "best at" in school. Where my expensive middle-class education went all wrong, that wilful emphasis on the subjective (or did it go right? is reading this worthwhile for you? ... am I perhaps an "author" after all?).

Well anyway, I'm doing art therapy in a blowy room in this all-too-open, chilly, 1940s-style mental ward. I write a few lines of the next instalment of *Poodle Play*, but my heart's not in it. I wander round the room. Everyone else seems so intent on what they're doing. One guy, who's older than his dyed-black hair and smart green suit imply, had gone to work at once. He's gathered together an incredible array of writing utensils: he's got coloured pencils, wax crayons, felt-tips, markers, ruler, india-rubber protrusion, protractors, even a compass. I look over his shoulder. He's drawing on turf-green sugar paper, designing what appears to be an airport. This isn't a fantasy about commercial holiday traffic at Heathrow, this is from the era when gentlemen took off in aeroplanes from tiny provincial air-fields to fight for their country. The precision of the drawing is terrifying: compass points, runway, position of wind sock, Lancasters "with twenty-five disposable bombs" (noted in black crayon alongside), bomb bay, control-tower, station for fire-engines.

I stare over the shoulder of the war veteran, then start my Mad imaginings. Straight into the psyche. Naked communion - none of that "sensible" crap - raw and direct, symbol-to-symbol. So I imagine goose-like flying-Vs of Messerschmitts ME-109s in the sky, primed to lay their explosive tonnage on the hospital: immediate terror, shaking cold-sweat fear. I'm running down the brown-lino hallway, nurses are alerted, I'm surrounded by both friends and foes, everyone arguing, laughing, shouting. Someone with a moustache I trust speaks to me, calms me down, makes me accept the coercion. I know where it'll go. It's so inevitable, so stupid. I let them take me down the corridor to a truly freaky room - all shiny with eighteenth-century pilasters, but with views across a valley dominated by pylons - and they tell me that drinking some rum-coloured, toxic noxion out of a plastic cup will "solve my problem." It won't, but I'm out-numbered. I drink the vile substance. When the NHS pays for it - no doubt some noble free-enterprise company needs to re-imburse its research costs - this draught of medicine probably costs twice as much as a bottle of champagne. But champagne for the oppressed would upset the petty satisfactions of the jobsworths and coupon-clippers. Mad Pride've got it right. This is a struggle about who gets what! "Normal" has nothing to do with it.

Not that they always give you knock-out drops. I drank the plummy draught, and was let go. I sauntered - in strangely elusive Pimpernel mode - out onto one of the brick-paved patios. Between suggestion and reality, a membrane had dissolved. Woodsmoke borne on the soon-to-die twilight wind. I laid down in one of the deckchairs, adjusting to its cool canvas curve. I suddenly craved the luxuriance of a cigarette, but contented myself with noticing the difference between the chill on my ankle and the post-medication warmth in my chest. Just like the swig of morphine-off-kaolin I shared with my cousin whilst staring at the passing trains between Gunnersbury and Kew Gardens in a never-to-be-forgotten, always to be re-invented, transgressive childhood. From the corner of one eye, I noticed a light going on in one of the upstairs rooms of my latest institutional confinement. To be breathing the night air and staring at an unconfined horizon, yet to be imprisoned! I allowed myself a nineteenth-century apostrophe.

The breeze is so cold, it blows right through my bones. I'm settling into deepfreeze autism ... but suddenly an angel appears before me. She's the new student nurse, she tells me, sent to get me to go to bed, but we can chat awhile. I can see she's intrigued but slightly alarmed to be talking to a genuine madman. I'm fascinated by her earrings. They're red and green, plaited glass strands. They symbolize Christmas, brightness, festivity, the gathering together of different ages. I tell her I'll go to bed. No point in antagonising the innocent. As I walk by the ex-airman, I ask him if I can have the drawing he's been working on. He says, "Sure!", and gives it to me. "I do 'em all the time. Usually just throw 'em away. You're welcome ..."

Later, sitting on my bed, I fold the A3 sugar-paper into eight parts, tear carefully along the folds. The pieces are a totem, a deconstructed map of evil scheming military genius. I keep it with an album I've taken from the hospital's collection of dodgy records, *Omniverse* by Fresh, on Prodigal Records. It's got a flying saucer on the cover in fetching retro-50s oils. Out of these fragments I can piece together all the predictable alien-invasion conspiracy shit (now that all this crap has gone mainstream, what have us lunatics got left? oh yes, that wise old mole, the revolution ...).

Still later, in London, "recovering from Madness," I use thin green cellotape to attach the pieces of the airport diagram to orange-coloured card (the colour so bright it still hurts my eyes). I write "IF FRIGHTENED GO FOR A SHIT" across it in colour-clashing red felt-tip, relaying some nurse's words of wisdom. Surrounded by the institutional white tile of the toilet you can feel safe. Even though they've got external keys to every "lock." It's scary as hell a lot of the time, being mad. Every sunset is a city burning on the horizon, every tree churning in the wind is a flight of robot magpies trained to peck out human eyeballs. Every sensation is so intense, it's like being reborn. Some kind of suffocating habit has been peeled off me, I'm raw and twitching, electrically sensitive. I never thought that going mad would be so *emotional*. Sobs welling up, hurting my chest, reminding me of childhood.

Take these slogans scrawled on an A4 file-pad sheet in dried-out red marker-pen:

ATTENTION!
Danny.

don't be feeling
guilty/swollen
heart like me.
fit to burst etc.
it was my *brother*
who taught me music.
want to meet him?

Panic attacks, the body writhing beneath the skin, complete confusion between emotional reactions and the effects of the medication. Later on, concerned doctors have me on drugs against the side-effects of the original drugs. The endless discussions about symptoms and side-effects and counter-drugs drive me crazy! The worse part of Madness is surely the technical aspects of "restoring sanity" (I only say that because the NHS is too underfinanced to give us any kind of extended consciousness-raising Freudian psychoanalysis. Such luxuries are impossibly expensive, darling! Give the poor suckers the old chemical truncheon instead ...).

But Madness really turns on the colours. Man! Sanity evidently survives in an unfocused, jellied miasma of black and white. Even now, leafing through these scraps, the sight of a red-purple envelope makes my heart race. Colour as a blinding invasion of the life-as-usual monotone. Whiff of scorched zinc. When I was mad and ecstatic, I used to think my heart would burst against my ribcage. I'd write in one colour, then write over it in another. Layers of meaning you could decode by playing different coloured lights upon the page. All the experiments with subjective vision Newton/Urizen never lets us make, preferring simply to enumerate the wave-lengths. Here's the back of a scrumpled, grey-white envelope. Big banner capitals hastily scrawled, the first three words in pale green, the rest in screaming red: "I'M JUST WRESTLING ... IT OUT OF YOU!" Over the top in black (graphite pencil): "I'M NO GURU ... YOU IDjut!" Mad statements always have a tendency to deploy extended techniques that cannot be reproduced in newsprint or ASCII text. Your senses five alerted - awake from the semiotic dream, bust the chain of signifiers! Why William Blake had to etch in copper-plate and print his own books - angels and demons skipping about his text. Colour-in each copy by hand or be lost to the abstract numerations of power and history.

Smells too! I remember dipping the corner of a letter in vanilla essence. Send the recipient a perfume bomb! Or cellotaping objects to the text, an end-of-pencil troll with long yellow nylon hair - give the postman a knobbly sensation as he handles the envelope. What's in there? A severed knuckle or what?

"I'M NO GURU": the usual schizo-Ratso Rizzo paradox, refusing both soapbox and pedestal, yet still shouting to be heard. "I'M JUST WREST-

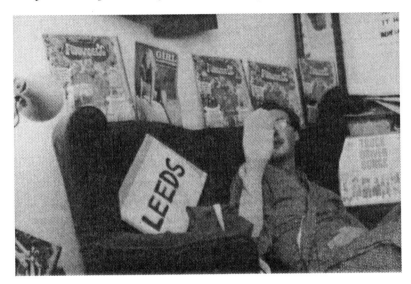

LING IT OUT OF YOU": the Latin root of education - *e-duco*, I lead out - it's not about sticking something in, it's about the immanent development of the taught. "IDjut" - punning the Freudian for your crazy greedy unsocialised babyself with the Irish pronunciation of "idiot." Watching James MacDougall at the Union Chapel doing a Johnny Rotten - not an imitation because he's doing the same thing, enacting the paradoxes of the anarcho non-leader, the schizoid seer. "Gotta get under the wall, off the stage, into the audience ... please don't be waiting for me!" Simon's photographing him: "Not just me!" Jim shoots back, "What about the others? They're here too, you know!" The messiah who tells us we're all sons of God, an anti-star to blackhole the entire fucking celebrity circus, implode the universe of social status. I'm not here anyway, I just stick around for my friends. You're not here either, of course. Self self, the perfect puzzle in the bourgeois carpet. The supercomplex braided knot that should be untied, unravelled into social threads. Flicking through these remnants from the stages of my fine fine superfine career in psychiatric illness, the last thing I want is for it to shed light on my individual soul. Why is it always flying saucers, Napoleon, Jesus, bombs, the

121

Queen Mother, fire engines, buses, the I.R.A., the Pope? If I could read this stuff as *social* documents, indications of a general malaise - attempts to flee the prison of my private, sane, limited, unhistorical and mortal existence - then they'd stop being sad and sordid and scary and deranged and become a field of play, as gleaming with lubricated release as a piece of Merz or a page of *Finnegans Wake* or a postcard from Ian Stonehouse or a tape from Dogbiz or a phone-call from Gamma. Name your poisson, fishface.

Isaac Newton split colour in a prism, measured degrees of refraction, decreed that the only lasting truth was held in unchanging laws specified by number. Johann Wolfgang von Goethe explored the effects of pressing fingers on closed eyelids, after-images, complementary colours that fringe any patch of intense coloration. Rebels and dreamers - from St Augustine to William Blake and William Burroughs - have always insisted on the projectile aspect of appearance, the images that manifest themselves during incipient sleep. Breaking through Newton's dualist metaphysics that divides eternal mathematical form from transient and insignificant matter or content, revolutionary materialism knows the sight of things moves nerves in the brain, impresses an indexical patterning whose return to the mind can be involuntary. For we are of the same stuff as the universe. Mind is not in another dimension from matter, it is what happens when matter becomes conscious of itself. The schizo pays attention to every refraction, refuses to dismiss any particle of thought or experience as "merely" subjective. The mauve echo of the flashgun on the iris is the imago of subjectivist militancy, the rebirth in new conditions of Kasimir Malevich's BLACK SQUARE.

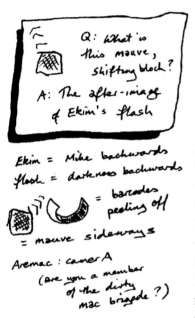

Q: What is this mauve, shifting block?

A: The after-image of Ekim's flash

Ekim = Mike backwards
flash = darkness backwards
= barcodes peeling off
= mauve sideways

Aremac : camerA
(are you a member of the dirty mac brigade ?)

I painted this sign and hung it above my array of *One Nation Under A Groove* gatefolds. Eyepopping commodity cartoon dayglo colours potlatching themselves to the retina, a bolshevik art assault on

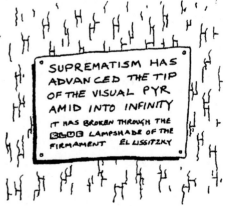

SUPREMATISM HAS ADVANCED THE TIP OF THE VISUAL PYRAMID INTO INFINITY IT HAS BROKEN THROUGH THE BLUE LAMPSHADE OF THE FIRMAMENT   EL LISSITZKY

the empyreal heavens. If it's all so predictable, if the psychiatrists and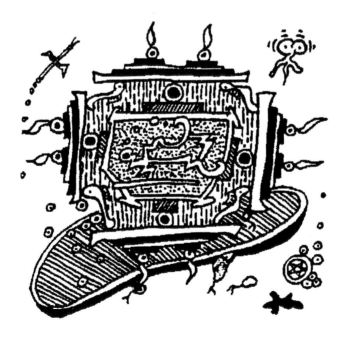
New Art History crumbsuckers have heard it all before, SO MUCH
THE BETTER. The possibilities and discontents of the capitalist order rub
shoulders in the interface between political revolt and subjective indulgence.
In their relentless war for profit, the capitalists drive our class into despair,
sickness, crime and madness; the revolutionary task is to seize these
fragments and weld them into weapons. Madness is not an individual failing
but a social hurt, caused by the suppression of a social possibility, the
egalitarianism and everything-for-everyone made possible by mass
production and digital technology. When the working class overturns the
property relations of capitalism - which, because it inflicts poverty and
starvation and war and boredom on us, we have every right to do - it is the
stockholders and captains of industry and generals and cops and politicians
and top artists and entertainers who shall "go mad." Reality will no longer fit
their concept of social reward and status. But, because they have bought into
anti-human ideologies of individual salvation and anti-social competition,
their madness will consist of nothing but psychosis, reaction, fascist revenge
on revolutionaries and refugees, mass death and uranium-depleted radiation
warfare. Unless our Madness - non-possessing, collective, anti-hierarchical:
social through and through - can win, the whole shebang is lost.

LEXICOGRAPHY
JAMES MACDOUGALL

We spend days before the TV set, sometimes too mesmerised even to make the short journey to the adjacent bedroom. Fucking knackering I think to myself, being unfortunate enough never to be able to switch off mentally. Unceasing words, thoughts and pictures, too awake to sleep, too depressed to stay alive.

I took the short walk to the village church last night for the mandatory ritual. Rubbing my cock against the cold granite gravestone, the hairs on the back of my neck stood to attention. In the process thoughts came and went, and the common alignments associated with day to day existence seemed somehow to disappear. Surrounded by the dark and cold, I felt so alive, psychic energy manifesting itself in the droplets of semen now resting on the epitaph and the surrounding grass. God, that was good I thought, quickly making a fast exit so as not to be seen. Another exercise executed with total self-gratification.

On the return route home, I stopped off at the off licence. Four cans of Special Brew later I fell into a deep sleep, the sort of sleep I crave. Looking at my bedside clock, 7:12am stared back at me. 14 hours out stone cold: great.

Thoughts of magic gurus have formed the basis of my mental landscape over recent days, culminating in a sort of friendly mental hell. Adjusting to the fact that I'm already possessed by darker forces, I try to remain vigilant so that they don't rise to the surface; fuck knows what would happen if they ever did. I've discovered through years of personal experience that devilish thoughts are best left ignored; that way, at least I can amuse myself without personal disaster.

I'd been allocated too many dirty chores to even care at the time of the murder. Usually well-mannered and polite, for some reason this night I snapped. All that the victim did was ask for a cigarette; true, hardly behaviour that warrants being murdered, but people can be so cruel and I'm only human, so fuck him. I took the cold-to-the-touch slab of meat and slowly drank the rich red blood that dripped over my chin and onto the floor below.

The attractive blonde on the bus home one day had basically been stalking me ever since. I felt it expedient to start up some sort of a rapport with her. "Turned out nice again." It was raining at the time. She stood and laughed, then invited me back to her apartment in the docklands for a glass of claret. Although quite plain looking herself, her apartment was lavishly decorated with matching furnishings and artefacts.

"That's an unusual vase you have on the mantelpiece," I told her.

"Oh that" she replied, "yeah, my father brought it back from Hong Kong. So, Jim..."

"What, Kate?"

"What do you do for a living? Finance? Stocks and shares, perhaps?"

"On the contrary, the majority of my time is spent visiting psychiatrists, watching cheap TV serials and very rarely eating."

"Oh I'm sorry, I didn't realise you were mad. I feel such a fool inviting you back under false pretences."

I was then shown the front door and told never to return.

Two days earlier, a member of staff had been given sick leave. I'd been trying to escape from my ward when the nurse in question gave hot pursuit.

"James, come back!"

James is the name that only a select few are permitted to voice. When other, less worthy individuals dare to use it, it just falls on deaf ears. Roy eventually caught up with me, and the pair of us crashed to the ground. Being extremely quick to get back on my feet, I was given - as if by an act of god - an ideal opportunity to fuck this cunt up. I must have kicked him hard, at least a dozen times in the face, head, ribs, kidneys and testicles, before the other members of staff had the chance to catch up and restrain me. If my memory serves me correctly - which it usually does - it took five of them to control my venom.

If the minister for health ever gets to read this: hello, I sincerely apologise for inflicting bodily harm upon one of your state nurses, and making him unfit for work for the eight weeks thereafter. Hopefully this unpleasant incident will never repeat itself.

The joys of a psychiatric lifestyle. All those pills to choose from, and learning to appreciate the sarcastic wit of the nurses. Fuck knows what went off last night: lots of shouting and crying from the cell next door. I'll ask Shutler after breakfast. He knew more about what was going on than the nurses did.

Shutler was a hard bastard, and responsible for the most violent vicious attack on Gerard Alexandra, the ward manager. It happened one day in the dining room. One has to remember that Alexandra was a nasty vindictive cunt whom nobody liked, and who was getting a bit too big for his boots. Well, until Shutler beat the living shit out of him that is. Oh, how we laughed.

"Here Shutler, do you know what went off last night?"

"Yeah, some bird got brought in during the early hours. Apparently she got raped while she was tripping."

"Poor cow, must've been a nightmare."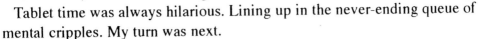

Tablet time was always hilarious. Lining up in the never-ending queue of mental cripples. My turn was next.

"I'll have six grams of smack, two eighths of whizz and a nice fat bag of crack please, nurse" I said, trying not to laugh.

"That's a bit inappropriate isn't it, James?" said the 19-year old student nurse in her thigh-hugging uniform.

"Can I fuck you, nurse?"

"Right, that's going in your report: sexually disinhibited language. You realise that you're not bringing forward your discharge prospects, with behaviour such as this."

"Big fucking deal. You read a poxy fucking text book and you think you're fucking Freud, you scheming little slut!"

After I said that, three other nurses crawled out of the woodwork and pinned me to the deck. A real treat that, being restrained and having a two-inch hypodermic stuck in my arse. Largactyl has the same effect of me as - if you can imagine - imbibing twelve cans of Special Brew and half a bottle of Martel brandy. It was a lot cheaper, and it meant that I could mong out in my cell for a couple of days.

It's Christmas eve today, and our ward has won the prize for the best-decorated; as if a bit of tinsel, a Terry's chocolate orange and a fairy could brighten the place up. This morning I awoke cold and bruised, wondering what the day had in store. It was a very violent place and every day, without fail, somebody would lose it. Today it was Neal's turn. I bumped into him in the corridor first thing, and he said that he was doing a runner to buy a bottle of vodka and that if anyone asked, I hadn't seen him.

The day drew on and nightfall was upon us. At about 10 o'clock four policemen walked in with Neal half-naked and bleeding profusely. The police seemed to be a bit on edge every time they came to the ward, this being no exception. Reg had had a seizure and Shutler had bitten off Dave's ear.

Christmas day, bored shitless, I decided to put on a fucked-up performance of the last supper for the nurses. I put all of the tables in the dining room in a horizontal line, then I sat in the centre in an ill-fitting ladies' night dress, stubbing cigarettes out on the palms of my hands - symbolic of the nails, you must understand - quoting paragraphs from *The Lion, the Witch and the Wardrobe*. They were not amused.

A new year, and the government apparently sits happily on its laurels. New Labour. New Britain. New? The same tired old theories day in day out, which only serve to make me gleefully and pointlessly look forward to my own fucking death. Lying on the psychiatrist's couch, openly masturbating as he takes some photographs for the Hiroshima hall of fame. I tell them I'm well. They beg to differ. I tell them I'm sick. They beg to differ. They tell me nothing that I don't already know as the psychopath hides in my mind's eye. I have to sit in a world of normal spastics. I admire your sanity; enjoy the rest of your life.

I was sitting in Hell last week, sipping from a freshly-squeezed glass of cum, shaken not stirred, no ice. Then, lo and behold, who should walk in but Death.

"All right Death, how's it hangin'?"

"Oh, y'know, surviving. I've just come across from the audit department to pick up an invoice for ten thousand fatalities this coming Tuesday."

"Do you enjoy your job?" I asked.

"Well, it's OK but the pay's shit. Have you seen Pestilence? I owe him a tenner."

"Nah sorry mate. Maybe he's up in Heaven talking to God."

"How long have you been condemned to Hell for?" he asked me, changing the subject.

"Oh, not long: four weeks."

"Pray tell me, what mortal sin did you commit, then?"

"I forgot to pay my television licence."

"Bastards. I'm of the opinion that television should only be used as a light source during fornication, and for keeping the children silent."

"Look out, here comes old Nick and he don't look too happy."

"Oh, don't worry about that. He's a very reasonable gentleman. Just a bit ugly, that's all."

He turned to Nick. "Nick, Jim and I were wondering if there were any chores that we could do for you. Maybe eat some shit, or perhaps fuck some dead children or animals?"

"Look chaps, things are getting pretty hot down here. I'm six months behind with the rent and the abyss agent has been threatening to cut my balls off and flush them down the fucking toilet!"

"Have you thought of re-inventing yourself as St. Lucifer and going back up to Heaven?"

"You're right. It's about time I retired!"

I put the boot in and the church door cracked open. There had been a remembrance service earlier that day and the stench of faith filled my nostrils. I walked up to the altar, rolled a joint and inhaled, lit the altar candles and started to undress. The rosary beads, the baby oil and the sacrificial dagger in my bag were to be the tools for this particular sex magick ritual. I got out the baby oil and rubbed it into my abdomen, temples and cock, rosary beads in one hand and dagger in the other. I then made a slight cut in the nape of my neck. The blood trickled down the blade.

I had to pick a sentinel. The photograph of the Princess of Wales seemed as good as anything. I looked at my watch. Five past midnight. The ritual began.

Rubbing the oil into my now fully-hardened cock, I could feel the winds of the earth moving across my back. The feeling was so intense that I now had to kneel. Faster and faster the thoughts came and went, from kicking out of the womb to the academy where I now sat with finely pointed fingers.

The surge of orgasm was upon me, clenching my cheeks and clearing my mind. I could feel the power from my kidneys moving up into the brain stem. Overpowered, the jissom shot from my throbbing cock all over the pile of pubes, blood, hair and the photograph. I laughed aloud as I noticed a letter of condolence, written by a six-year old girl, attached to the photo and I used that to clean my cock. Leaving the church dowsed in petrol, I lit the Zippo and threw it into the pile of prayer books. If there was a God he would live in Paris and catch the Metro bus to the coast.

PSYCHOSIS AS A REVOLUTIONARY WEAPON

MICHAEL HOWLETT

As the cherubs of repose dollop your brow with the puckered promise of the world of dreams, and the lateness of the hour devours your extremities with the needlings of an empire away from the everyday, gather up your final gram of resistance and scrub the slumber from your sockets. Grapple with this base instinct which keeps you in synch with the square world and get ready to vent your violence when we vanquish "sleep, which is the greatest thief, as it steals half one's life."

Sleep is a coma, a death-like state, which people pull willingly over themselves like a blanket, and it is to myself and my learned colleagues a reprehensible condition which must be obliterated.

TIPS FOR FIGHTING SLEEP'S DEATH-LIKE GRIP:

1. THE INTENT - While society sleeps, bound to this archaic ritual, we shall take over.

2. THE DRINK - The dewy drops of perspiration from another's brows, flavoured as they are with the mania of the long in waking.

3. THE MANTRA - "KILL, KILL, KILL FOR INNER PEACE AND MENTAL HEALTH!"

4. THE SARTORIALS - Pyjamas, once clownish and babylonian, now present themselves as a bold new uniform for the army fighting against the nauseous prospect of the ethical workday, and also as a salute to madness and possibility - both children of the night sky.

Deny yourself the rituals which coincide with sleep's preparation. Do not wipe the taste of the day away with the false and foreign taste of mint, but relish the compacted and compounded evidence of an evening well spent!

JUST SAY NO TO TOOTHPASTE!

A VISION OF ELVIS
LUTHER BLISSETT

I was posing with my slave for the wankers taking photographs on the other side of the hospital gates.

"Say cheese" I said, giving my slave a whack round the chops, "they'll fuck off in a minute."

"Wouldn't you rather be somewhere else?" he whined.

"Not at all!" I snapped. "The oxygen of publicity is my life's blood!"

The cunts standing on the pavement in Homerton High Street clicked away relentlessly on their cameras, hoping that at least one of the shots would turn out halfway decent. Lisa, my key nurse, chucked a handful of confetti into the air, which would look wicked in the photographs. Just like snow. Know what I mean?

In my hand I held an old tobacco tin which contained the answers to life, the universe and everything. I stroked it furtively, turned, and gave my slave a swift right hook to the kidneys. He responded by doubling up in agony and coughing up one third of a pint of brown, lumpy substance.

Once I had a dream. I'd been sitting quietly listening to one of His records. A brief encounter, that was all. He couldn't quite understand what He was doing up in heaven. He was fretting, as if He had a heavy weight on His shoulders. Tired old fears about whispers and rumours, even up in heaven.

I hit my slave with a karate chop to the windpipe, and that relaxed him a little.

There was a time in ancient Egypt when people built huge tombs. I don't suppose we'll ever know why they bothered.

My slave took the tobacco tin from my hand, knelt before me and proceeded to undo my flies. "You can have whatever you want," he simpered. He was ever so sweet.

Before long he'd liberated my stiffening cock from the bounds of decency and was alternately chewing, sucking and swallowing greedily on the raw meat while the photographers snapped away. To increase my sense of arousal I pinched his nostrils shut and watched him asphyxiate, and it wasn't long before I deposited one third of a pint of liquid genetics down the back of his throat just in time before he passed out.

The hospital had been built in the good old days. Decrepit as it was, it had a certain kind of charm: a faded, wasted sort of glory, falling splendidly apart at the seams. It was a perfect day as I zipped myself up and strolled back to the ward. I'd never enjoyed a day better. In fact, I might even have gone so far as to say that it was really quite nice considering.

They brought my slave to me on a stretcher and he soon came round. After binding his hands and wrists, then gagging and blindfolding him, I tired of his company and walked around the ward deciding which of the nurses to shag this time.

The chandeliers suspended from the nicotine-stained ceilings were all that remained of the glory of days gone by at the Hackney Hospital. As I gazed upwards, I fantasised about the days when photo-shoots would be unnecessary to secure my future well-being.

My slave reflected upon the ephemeral nature of my success.

"When all this is over" he bleated, do you think we'll know what 'love' means?"

"Not if I can help it!" I spat. "Anyhow, I don't know what you're talking about. Change the subject at once!"

Lisa arranged for the pictures to appear in the Hackney Gazette the next morning, along with a story headlined: "TOP ROCK STAR LOSES IT AND GETS LOCKED UP IN LOCAL BIN." The story suggested that there was something improper about the lifestyle I was allowed to lead whilst detained on one of her majesty's sections. I didn't give a fuck. Since promising to marry the medical director as soon as they let me out, I'd been given the run of the place.

The memory of the visitation by The Dead Elvis Presley had troubled me a little. The accounts I gave of the event, to people who were little more than strangers, prompted the prescription of a medication which did very little to stimulate my senses. In fact, it suppressed all flights of the mind until at times I rather resembled a zombie. And yet stubbornly I continued to tell my story, until my record company arranged for me to be carted off to hospital, to shut me up.

The hospital blankets were decorated with far too many blim holes to pass for class, but they kept us warm. I usually kept the tobacco tin under my pillow while I slept: it contained the secrets of love, pain, fear, sex and death; and when awake I lit scented candles. During the daytime, the sun filtered through the institutional gold lame curtains and the smoke haze, making it much lighter than it was at night. On the beanbag on the other side of the room, Lisa kept us under close observation while searching through her pockets to make sure that the cocaine was still there.

"The boss says you'll have a CD out next week, collecting together all three of your EPs" the nurse commented. I suspect that she may have been a plant from the record company. "Then you'll be performing a concert to promote it at the Jolly Butchers in Stoke Newington."

"How the fuck will I get there?" I scoffed, "I'm on a fucking section!"

"We'll organise some escorted leave," she explained.

"Shut up and chop us some lines, bitch!" I commanded.

She did as he was told, and after snorting one of the lines she passed the mirror to me. I took a toot and then passed it along to my slave.

"I love the photo they printed in the Hackney Gazette," he twittered.

"What, the one with the snow?"

"No, the one of me sucking your knob."

That night, for the first time ever, I told my slave about the visitation from The Dead Elvis Presley.

"I've met Elvis!" I boomed.

"Me too!" he ejaculated.

"No you haven't!" I challenged him.

"Yes I have!" he insisted. "He's a bit blacker than you might expect, but he's alive and well and living in Hackney!"

"It must be a different Elvis then," I countered.

"Yeah?"

"Yeah!" I affirmed, poking him viciously in the ribcage with a snooker cue. "When I met Elvis I was resting in bed, mid-afternoon, having a wank, listening for the first time to *How Great Thou Art* as sung by The King Of Rock 'N' Roll Himself, when the kitchen door opened ever so slightly, gently, and I felt... A presence! He floated in as if I were an old friend, and just started talking to me! He sat recounting some of the terrible things He'd done with his time here on this earth, and wondering what the fuck He was doing up in heaven. So I did my best to reassure Him. "Don't worry!" I said. I insisted that He needed to snap out of it and enjoy being up there. He should just relax, pull His socks up and get on with it. I'd probably have said the same to anyone to be honest with you, but it seemed to do the trick. And then, as quickly as He came, He went. He was a perfect gentleman. The door opened ever so slightly again, and then He was gone. I lit a spliff and carried on listening to the record."

My first big international hit *Five 'A' Sides* on Rather Records had recently been revived on the West End night club circuit, causing a thrilled reaction from the kids. It seemed that my 'file under cult obscurity' days were over. The money from the royalty cheques, together with my DLA and incapacity benefit, added up to a decent wedge. I was rich!

I had a vision of the apocalypse and told my slave about it.

"If everyone farting and dying is filling the air full of methane, and all that stuff is going up into space and just floating there, above and beyond the hole in the ozone layer, and if someone lit a match or sent a nuclear missile and it exploded, would the earth become like another sun? I mean, I saw these two suns burning brightly."

Breakfast was Weetabix washed down with red wine. After breakfast it was late evening and time for the show, so my slave and I got dressed and we were driven to the Jolly Butchers in an ambulance.

On the way in the bouncer called me to one side. "Here's your rider" he whispered, handing me the sheet of blotting paper surreptitiously.

"Thanks mate," I winked back at him, smacking my slave around the side of the head with the mikestand I'd been carrying.

The bouncer gave me a funny look. "You're not going to take that all at once, are you?" he asked me.

"Of course not" I lied as I waltzed through the door. At the bar my bass player passed me a joint laced with cocaine and I sucked on it greedily while the barmaid fixed me a bloody mary to wash the tabs down with.

"My fucking arse is sore" my slave complained, "it's because your cock's so huge!"

This statement seemed to excite a perfectly pleasant gentleman standing within earshot. After twenty seconds of conversation I led him into the dressing room and allowed him to kneel before me and unzip my flies. My cock sprang into action immediately and I wasted no time in ramming the raw meat right down the back of the bloke's throat. As I did so, the acid kicked in and the doors of perception flew open. I can truly say that I felt at one with all the living creatures that roamed the earth as my groupie's neck muscles strained tightly around my marauding spam javelin. Before long it felt as if all of the planet's oceans were emptying into the gentleman's throat, when in fact, it was merely one third of a pint of liquid genetics flowing from one living creature to another.

The next day, I couldn't remember the rest of the evening, but the Hackney Gazette reported that the gig was shite, and it appeared that my slave had been admitted to an intensive care ward with multiple fractures. The CD didn't sell as well as hoped, the royalties dried up, and when I was discharged from hospital I broke my promise to marry the medical director. She really wasn't my type.

I found out later that soon after, Lisa woke up one morning in a drug sweat frenzy having had only four hours' sleep. The balance of her mind felt disturbed by ultra-vivid dream experiences which told her something she couldn't quite understand. She walked into the bathroom and had a good long look at herself in the mirror. She washed, shaved, brushed her teeth and combed her jet-black hair into a quiff. While swigging from

a bottle of Hundred Pipers and polishing her boots, she decided to go
to Memphis: she had to go to Memphis! She packed a bag with a
couple of pairs of leather trousers, some clean knickers and a fine selection
of silk shirts. She wrote a farewell note, got her passport and put it in the
inside pocket of her tuxedo jacket. And as she walked out of the hospital for
good she blew a kiss behind her.

This was all a while ago. These days I live in a community residential unit
for retired rock stars, where recently I had one final vision, or visitation. I
was listening to *How Great Thou Art* as sung by The King, when I saw two
suns melt into one, as in the lid being placed onto a tobacco tin. Elvis had
witnessed the contents of the tin: Old Holborn. Two suns became as one, and
because I'd absolved Him, I knew that He was OK now.

MENTAL
CHRIS P.

My game of mental ping-pong grew more complex. My opponent and me were equally flexed, it was only slight lapses in concentration that let me through with a sucker punch. We was both focused on a fresh game plan. In our mind's eye we sent that twinkling ball back and forth like some boss rap between MCs. My opponent tried to stop access into their court with hard floor tactics and some well def obstacles. I attempted to stop the shimmering symbol access into the area of my phunky psyche. In the trad form, time passed and sweat dripped from my face. The path of hairlessness ain't always slickest. Salt stung my peepers and the globe wove its way through my underground maze. My reply was allied with a megablast mind monster. Hey, all's fair when you're a bad young brother. I caught an edge of panic from my opponent, then it was me who was back on guard. Suddenly our game of mental telepathy was shattered. One of our number must have been well damaged to make such a mental outburst.

Our game disappeared in a blaze of white light and I was left holding my head in my hands. The pain was flowing wild style, but smoky, silky fingers of comfort quickly met my brain. I sent out my own feelers and all of us began to chill. The spasm passed. Making mass contact, the whole was not complete. A part of us had gone and I shivered with more than just a cold sweat. A piece of our pie had been baked. A form seemed to be present, but there was a mental space where before it had been possible to communicate on another level. Speaking without words is whack but takes time. It's maximum skill to put experiences, feelings, ideas and desires into a transmissible form. It's a fool's move to think that you can just open your mind and let someone else into it. Hey, not even all my loud and proud notions are available in total recall. When I'm on my own I get the chance to check out the corridors of my own mind, stumbling on misplaced moments and hidden artefacts that take me back. My exposure to outside forces has been limited lately due to my ruffneck confinement, but my four white walls means I can investigate my new jack mind skills.

In the beginning I could only detect the hard knocks and the illumination confused the shit outta me. Where was this hype at and why was I receiving it? I slowly came to develop a system as signals came from other sources. Some tones were soothing, but others contained anger louder than bombs. With time our group got more sussed and I became more chilled, though maybe this had something to do with my medication. I began to make up some wicked looks for the others I could hear in my head. I invented my own faces for them since I couldn't meet them live and direct.

Sometimes I wondered if this was some total hype flavour bugging my brain, but the voices had characters and emotions that was way off of my style big time. There were six other bodies of thought I caught communications from. No names though, so no incriminations. Sorted.

My diagnosis by the shrinks was paranoid schizophrenia and when I took my medication it took me far, far away. No way could I engage in mental antics when drugged to the eyeballs on the shit they gave me. I could never tell the nurses about the cool phatness in my head. They weren't believers, and conversation with these suckers was always a waste of time. My mind don't depend on a whacked vocab. When I'm flowing I can feel a breeze and erase the debris in the dark corners. Let the juice loose. The concern now was why as a whole we was only six when we was seven. The scat, slim, erratic sounding voice no longer kicked in with the fairy tales told to them when they was young. We never heard the sound of sleep that night.

After the morning slop had been forced down my throat and I'd hidden my pills under my tongue before grounding them into powder under my feet, I resumed contact with the (tele)pathic posse. Access to my fellow loonies was limited since I was considered a danger after whopping that sick shits ass one more time. The story goes that big Bill had been given a lobotomy yesterday. Without warning he was taken away and given an incision straight into the frontal lobe of his brain. The doc certainly made Bill into a flower pot man. He must have been the missing member of our silent world. Paranoia kicked in as I wondered if this meant that the docs in the loony bin were after stopping all the telepaths rappin.

Maybe it was always to be so. Authority suppresses what it is afraid of and does not understand. This was the deal so they could cover their asses and preserve their position of power. This train didn't stop at their station, so maybes they was trying to terminate it early. If this was a step forward it was one step beyond for the powers of control protecting the status quo. The sounds from the underground may be a danger, so wipe them out early. I guess this is what brought us nutters into the predicament we found ourselves in. Shit, I'd been that scared I'd brought myself in. Now it seemed they weren't happy on letting me out again. There weren't no care in the community, so instead of their patience I was stuck as some sucker patient in their mental asylum. For real.

It was tough to keep my violent streak in check when I could catch a sneak peek at some stranger's thoughts when they walked on by. If they was dissing me then I lashed out at them. It happened inside here n'all since some of the hired musclehead attendants weren't much more than boot boy thugs who enjoyed kicking my skinny ass off the walls. That last time I'd got them back was when the screws between my fingers from the window frames drew red, red blood. And I'd kinda been hoping it woulda been black like tar. It was how their insides seemed like to me anyway. After that stunt I was stuck in the solitary sin-bin. I guess they supposed this would do my head in big time, but I welcomed the break. I could focus on the forces going off in my head and sort my shit out. The glass of muddy water in my mind separated and the silt sank to the bottom. I meditated on my glass of sugary liquid and came to the conclusion I liked it here. I was in the place to be. Right now I never even had to concern myself with the everyday concerns of the suckers outside. I was catching that train to other mental planes.

I communicated with the deep, all embracing waves of thought emitting from way over to my left. They too believed the governors of the institution were after wrecking the telepath party. Don't get caught seemed to be the name of this game. I made a mental note to modify my behaviour so they all would swallow that insane shit and avoid that power kick. I did a little shit picture in my cell that afternoon to keep them happy. Smearing my own crap on the walls was a new one for my file. It'd keep them bastards guessing anyhow. My war of wits became the actual fact soon enough. The evening of my whacked shit hit, there was another blinding outburst in my head. This megablast was worse than the last. The blood about my brain pulsed with too much pressure and my mind ached. Deep, embracing had left the building. I felt trashed and mashed and feared the implied revelations. Someone was tracking down the voices I spoke to in my head and winding up the stunt. The ability was breaking up between us.

The next day the deep, embracing voice was revealed to me to be a sister called Victoria suffering from bulimia. She'd ended up in this nut house as a result of an eating disorder. Vicky had had a shock, literally as the volts which were meant to fix her messed with her mind. Who are the sick fucks who come up with this shit is what I want to know. Our uniqueness was being annihilated and it was difficult keeping cool when contacting the others. I didn't know what to do with my body, so I got down by getting under my bed to try and avoid getting the fear. Despite the contact with the (tele)pathic posse I felt very alone. Mental tendrils of sympathy can be soothing, but I couldn't even remember the last time I was hugged. I cracked and cried myself into something that sometimes seemed like sleep.

Fuck, the morning came with one big boom. There were three of them in my cell with a warning for me for not using the lavatory. With my mattress over me they proceeded to kick the shit outta me. You watch too many cop shows for real to believe this crap will mean the bruises won't show. This wasn't the physical contact I'd had in mind previously. I laid low, braced myself and let them go about their bizness. From my position under the mattress I could still scan their auras in full effect. They made for depressing viewing. Channel zero in the land of panic is mostly made of nicotine-stained and lager-soaked guilt, stress, worry, doubt and incomprehension. I could even smell a sort of fear, and hey, what if I did almost feel sorry for their domestic barnies, money worries and social inadequacies? I knew there was no way I could dwell on their way, so I rocked the funky beat and brought the noise.

I was hit with a flash and remembered my childhood. I was in the playground with my foster mother when I fell from the climbing frame and hit my head. I was out like a light for less than a minute, but I was sure I floated above my body while a white light flooded my senses. I went back to my body and not into the tunnel of light, but the impression of this memory was a bolt out of the blue. C'mon and bring your skills to the battle. Warning the four other presences in my world to shield themselves, I faked a mental orgasm on the darkside. Shit happens and then some. This free-style thought had some sonic soul force and I hoped I'd bugged my oppressors' minds good. The boots on my back stopped a moment and I bolted. Suckers had left the door open so I closed it on them as I legged it out the place. I wasn't looking back, just for some way out and my style was wild. My speed carried me from danger down corridors and toward the fire escape. Smashing the bar back I realised it hadn't been padlocked shut with a chain. Phunky cold sweat of fate.

Stepping down metal steps to a well wet playing field below felt like entering some new garden. From here I'd heard that there was a gate which backed onto the canal path. I said a little prayer for the late workers at the institution, they sometimes left it open. Again the main mixman was smiling and I stole the right to fight straight through the gate. Still nothing stirring at the loony bin so I was good and gone.

I flinched as I felt another presence but the mister with the dog collar laid out his own phrase. "Do not be afraid, my son," Priest-man says, "I had a dream that I would meet someone today who would need saving."

I said nothing, but thanked him telepathically and he smiled. I attempted to put some notion into his head about him letting me check out his joint.

"Please, would you do me the favour of accompanying me to the vicarage? I can feed and shelter you whilst you choose your next direction."

I grinned as I caught this fly tip outta here, I wasn't going to rot fenced in. This sucker thinks he has me, I know I can shut him down. Word.

NO HANGOVERS IN HEAVEN
TED CURTIS

I had been out of the Maudsley for about three weeks following a six-month stretch spent there for the kidnapping of my next-door neighbour's dog, Sid, which seemed to bark incessantly and piss in the lift all of the time, and also at irregular hours. I'd immediately cashed six months worth of DLA cheques amounting to about £1750, having gone home only once just before dawn to collect my passport and a few clothes, and I had then fled the country, getting the daily bus to Dublin which leaves Victoria at around 8 am.

I feared the wrath of my neighbours, a pair of drug-dealing hippie brothers who had lived on the estate all of their lives. Whilst it wasn't a particularly rough estate, I had often heard them fighting with their girlfriends in the wee small hours and I feared for my future. I had returned the dog alive but I had cut out its tongue with some embroidery scissors that I kept in the kitchen drawer, ostensibly for opening bags of coffee and orange juice cartons with a bare minimum of mess. Whatever you may have heard in court, I love animals and my mother very much. I would have liked to have done the same thing to the hippie brothers, and worse things still to their wailing women, but the price of this was simply too high.

Somewhat bleary-eyed having been on the vodka spritzers for all of the previous day, with my irises bloodied from the habitual rubbing of those same eyes which comes with the perennial combination of hangovers and insomnia, I alighted at the terminus that is Dublin bus station. I don't normally drink a great deal, but I hadn't been able to renew my amitryptyline and procyclidine prescriptions in time for the bus trip and I had been getting the shakes and the odd side-vision. The journey over from London by coach and boat takes a total of twelve and a half hours, and during this vodka-popping daydreaming head-time a plan began to take morph on the inside of my head.

Over the past few months it had emerged that the socialist establishment were tabling what had been termed by some as 'the mental health act from hell', some of the more extreme provisions of which made forced treatment over the cornflakes look like the teddy bear's picnic. I could only suppose that they were national socialists or something, being a national government. I had also heard on the early news that a small cabinet grouping, minus Tony Blair, was travelling to Dublin for a peace process pow-wow in only two days' time. Clearly, something had to be done.

I singled out Alan Milburn, the new health minister, Jack Straw, the inappropriately-monikered Joseph Goebbels looky-likey, Peter Mandelson, the real power behind the throne, Alastair Campbell, the PR guru and former pornographer, and David Blunkett, who I just hated anyway: he was the worst fascist of the bunch, but because of his own disability most people were afraid to have a go at him and he always managed to avoid any real flak. I wasn't even sure what he was even doing there at all; perhaps he had just got lost or something. The Queen Mother was also flying in separately to give the whole fiasco her personal blessing. I seemed to be the only person who knew that she had died and had been replaced with an android in 1973. Once, after one of her so-called 'hip operations' (cool Britannia!), I had waited outside of the Harley Street hospital where she had been treated with the rest of the crowds. When she had emerged, I had turned on my mobile phone and watched as her head bobbed uncontrollably from side to side and she began turning a rapid pirouette with her metal legs at 90-degree angles to one another. She was swiftly bundled into the back of a waiting Daimler, her face at the window replaced with an emergency cardboard cut-out incorporating a hand on a spring that waves like one of those nodding dogs from the seventies. But I digress. In only 48 hours, I had to plan their demise and my swift escape, and find the necessary hardware. It would be tough going. Then I dozed off for a bit.

After getting off the bus and changing over a couple of hundred pounds inside the bus station, I made my way nominally north-west over onto Lower Gardiner Street, opposite the big roundabout that faces the Custom House. Having stayed there before, I instinctively knew where I was heading: the Cedar Manor youth hostel.

The sultry post-youth who answered my ringing at the hanging-off doorbell of the place was familiar to me, if not I to him. A somewhat taciturn fellow, he merely rolled his eyes and eyebrows up at me from looking down at his clipboard, anticipating my request for accommodation without even the least of his characteristic mutterings that I remembered so well from the last time.

"Um, yeh. I need a single dorm bed for about three days, probably. Do you need that all up front?"

"Ah, yuh-yuh" he mumbled, rubbing at the side of his nose like a bored refugee from some late-period Charles Bukowski poem.

"Cash?"

"Ah, yeh" he informed me. I handed him £30 and he scribbled out something illegible onto the top page of a non-carbonned receipt book and handed it grubbily over to me, together with three pound coins. I noticed that he had also scrawled the security-code and dorm numbers for the room downstairs onto the reverse of the tatty remnant. After only a year or two spent away, I was familiar with the drill. You never forget your first bicycle ride nor either your first night in jail, as they say.

Staying in the cheapest accommodation that you can find in one of

144

the most beautifully historical city centres in the world is not something quickly forgotten. I recalled immediately the missing tiles on the shower floors and the hot water that never came, the boys from the north of the country and the way that they took up semi-permanent residence in the television room from 6 pm onwards, and how they sneered at the English guests and barely tolerated the rich American New-Englanders there. On the sign out front it proudly said 'Backpacker's Hostel', but half of those there were down from Derry and Antrim for the labouring work up the hill. I felt like telling them about the suffering and the crippling poverty in ethnic Somerset, but it wasn't my place. The madness of King Henry the Eighth had a lot to answer for. The combined madnesses of Straw, Milburn, Campbell, Mandelson and Blunkett, along with princess Elizabeth the deceased, were soon to redress the balance with their insipid German blood, only of course they didn't know that yet. Only I did.

The following day, having set my alarm for 8 am I sprang up immediately and went to take the obligatory freebie shower. I was just getting the strawberry soap between me buttocks when I heard a voice calling me.

'Ted! Ted!' it intoned. I looked up at the shower-head, but the voice had moved to just behind my left shoulder, the one that I had put out whilst chasing Sid the bad puppy around the back of my television sets. 'Ted!' it told me again.

"Go on," I said. "I'm waiting."

'Tara can tell you where to get everything that you need. You know, *Tara!*'

"And?" I waited. But there were no more replies. Suddenly sensing that time was even more now of the essence, I abandoned the washing of my feet and I got out of there.

Back in my dorm, somebody was rolling over in his cot and farting. I hurriedly changed into the same old dirty clothes and then I dashed up the stairs to ground level. I rushed past the kitchen, at this hour stacked to the brim with those chatty builder's labourers. Once I was past the deserted reception desk, I next found myself charging headlong down Gardiner street and left towards Busaras.

The hill of Tara in county Meath was the site for the gathering of the Irish High Kings from the 1st century up until around the 6th, and then for the Kings of Leinster right up until the 11th: and of Brian Boru, perhaps the greatest of these, who finally sent those Vikings packing on their longboats from Clontarf back in the sixties or something. Later still, it was site for Daniel O'Connell's biggest ever gig in 1843. Many people consider it to be a mystical place still, and buses run there regularly. Suddenly I knew where I was going. I walked up to the information kiosk in Busaras, glad that I had thought to pick up my shoulder bag with some money in it on my way out, and still trying to find my breath.

"Talla," I exclaimed through the filthy perspex screen. "Tawwap!"

"I'm sarry?"

Fortunately it was still early in the morning and there was not too much of a queue behind me. I paused, screwed up my eyes, looked groundwards and pinched my nose for a bit. Then I looked up again.

"Tara," I tried again. "A bus to the hill of Tara?"

"Well, there's the guided tour, that's £13. Leaves in an hour and a half and you'll be back for tay. Or you could just get the number 63 to Drogheda and change: it'll be cheaper for ye."

"That sounds good. How long would I have to wait for the connection?"

She pushed a photocopied bus timetable to me through a small gap at the bottom of the screen, and I scanned across it as I picked it up. Other than having to go through Drogheda and Navan, the bus didn't take very long. There was one in twenty minutes. I wasn't bothered about the cost of the fare: this appeared to be my destiny! If it came to it then I could always hawk my passport and my bus ticket back to London.

"Thanks very much!" I told her.

"Thanks so."

And purposefully, I made off towards the Eason's mini-shop. I needed a newspaper to check for political developments, and also a phone card in case I felt like making any threatening calls.

The bus journey went particularly well in the winter sunshine, and by high noon I was walking alongside the base of the mighty hill. Although anybody is free to just stroll up its sides, I thought that that I might save my legs and skirt the bottom for about an hour. If by then I had still not been contacted, either from afar or perhaps from somewhere nearer, I would attempt some semblance of an ascent. After about half an hour of ambling around its perimeter smirking bright-eyed into the sun, I heard a whispering from all around.

'Ted!'

"Y'ello!"

'Ted!'

"Mmmm..."

'Are you sure that you can do this?'

"Yeh."

'You want the Jonathan Swift exhibition. It's been kept on until December 14th.'

"Anything else?"

Silence.
"Allo?"
More of the same.

Sitting down in the bus station waiting-room at Drogheda, I scanned through the listings magazine that had come tucked inside of the 'Irish Independent' that I had purchased back in Dublin. It was Thursday. Scanning through the 'exhibitions' section on page 29, I ascertained that the Jonathan Swift show had indeed been kept on until December 14th, and that it was in the foyer of the National Library, which adjoins Leinster House where the Dail meets. Satisfied that I was one step further in my momentous mission, and with forty minutes remaining to wait for my connecting bus, I made my way outside. Now I don't know whether or not there is all that much to Drogheda other than the obvious history, but if there is then I've never seen it. All that I have seen is a large coach park, a small waiting room, and a road with a drive-by McDonald's opposite. This was where I was now heading.

When I got there I found the door locked against me, with a large poster facing outward from the inside stating 'Closed for a radical rethink on the future of the planet'. I blinked hard, and when I opened my eyes again it said instead, 'Closed due to food poisoning'. Still desperate for a snack or for something to kill the remaining time, I noticed a nearby waste bin. I had a root through it and found, amongst a few empty crisp packets and coke cans, a rather heavy blue plastic carrier bag. When I pulled it out I found to my astonishment that it contained a snub-nosed Uzi 9mm machine pistol.

'Told ye!' a voice behind me said, but when I looked around there was nobody there. I hurriedly stuffed the thing into my shoulder bag and deposited the carrier bag back inside the waste bin, where it landed with a thud that was heavier than that which one might expect from an empty sack. Having quickly retrieved it, I found that I had almost missed three spare ammunition magazines and a half-bottle of Jameson's.

The next morning I rose early again, took my free shower and didn't bother to check out properly, so that I wouldn't have to lug my rucksack around with me as well. Let the fuckers sweat, I thought to myself. That was what *I* had been doing all night in a twelve-berth dormitory, trying to sleep with a machine-gun under my pillow. I spent the morning murdering time in the municipal art gallery and the writer's museum on Parnell Square, before making my way down Parnell Street and then south to a nice little eaterie that I knew of near to the corner of Mary Street. There I took in a baked potato and some fortifying coffee. I was saving the whiskey for the next day.

Carousing east, the christmas decorations were strung across the street at above head height with a vengeance, and radio speakers hung from them playing seasonal tunes and occasional news bulletins. "The murder trial continues today of a 56-year old County Roscommon farmer who shot dead his eight-year-old son on account of his excessive drinking," the newsreader informed busy shoppers and wayward drifters alike. I bought myself a couple of nice pens, a single biro, a cigarette lighter and an A4 pad in the Eason's further along Mary Street, which is also quite a good place to go for greetings cards if you're interested, and I stuffed them surreptitiously into my bag in the crowded street outside, taking care not to open it up too widely. I walked down across O'Connell Bridge and made for College Green and an academic bookshop, still open for business just before the end of term. Once inside I made straight for the literature section and selected Swift's complete poems, and then a rather chunky volume on eighteenth century Dublin and its notable luminaries. This was to be my cover: surely no student of poetry would appear to want to bump off David Blunkett with his witty turns of phrase, I thought to myself. The resulting package proved rather bulky so I decided to carry the bag separately, heading for Kildare Street and my final destination.

It was by now 1 pm and I bought the £3 day reader's ticket. I thought that I might have to leave my passport at the door, but instead they just wrote down the serial number and not even my name. I spent the afternoon perusing Swift's observations and witticisms in verse. He was really very funny in places, and once or twice I found myself having to bite down on my lower lip so as not to draw attention to myself. The historical tome was also fairly revealing, making a bit of a change from A Star Called Henry and Cecil Woodham-Smith's The Great Hunger. To complete the picture, I found the appropriate bookshelves and pulled down Daniel Defoe's Journal of the Plague Year, Maria Edgeworth's Castle Rackrent and a related volume on architectural styles. Then, at just a little after four o'clock, I waited for a slight bit of activity and it came: I gathered up my things, leaving just a black biro behind, and I pretended to go off for the restrooms. I found that just past these and off to the right, there lay a secluded boiler room. I made to settle in for the night.

Finding my way out later from the boiler room, up a spiral staircase and then across a slight roof space and into the central welcoming chamber of Leinster house, lit only by a fag lighter which kept on burning my thumb, was no mean feat, but I had come a long way baby, as they say, and so I persevered. Once properly in I located a closed-off viewing gallery where they evidently had the painters and the plasterers in. Well, that's handy I thought, and I hauled myself up there to sleep.

The next thing that I heard was a series of voices coming from the central chamber, and I knew that I had not been detected.

'*It is time!*' a Spanish accent informed me from an empty pot of sunshine-yellow undercoat. I pushed my glasses up onto my nose and, squinting, I retrieved the gun and the cartridges from my bag. I pulled out a mobile phone from my coat with my left hand, dialling 121 and pressing the 'call' button, and I quietly placed it up on the hand railing of the viewing gallery.

As operator services began to list interminable options, the Queen Mum suddenly turned through 540 degrees, went careering into the nearest wall and promptly exploded in a sheet of flame, setting some fire-retardant curtains alight. I got up onto one knee to beg for death, aimed, and blew out the main chandelier. Peter Mandelson screamed and then he began singing 'SOS' by Abba. Jack Straw looked around through his bottle-bottoms for a baby to snatch and shield himself with, but none were available. I took aim again and his head came off and he was gone. Mandelson was now dancing: I pointed the gun at him and took his legs off, leaving him to bleed to death. Blunkett had jettisoned his dog and was heading for the nearest fire escape, the truth revealed. The sprinkler system had kicked in and sirens were going off everywhere. It was chaos. I drew myself up to my full height, leaned over the balustrade and screamed "NOW YOU DIE!!" I shot Blunkett about fourteen times through the back just as he got the door to the fire escape open, and his dog ran around him, saliva drooling and harness dragging.

Then I saw the real minister of propaganda, Alastair Campbell, cowering behind a speaker's rostrum with an armed-and-jacketed Garda sergeant crouching by his side and taking aim at me. He let fly as I moved to the right and winged me in the left shoulder, bringing back the old jip there, but as he did this Campbell stood up smirking and I severed his head at the neck in a flurry of spent cordite fumes. I crouched back down again, put another magazine into the shooter and, pulling aside a dust sheet, I saw the faceless Geordie fascist Alan Milburn heading for Blunkett's cadaver at the fire escape. But luck was not with him: Blunkett's dog leapt up and slobbered over his face and I completely destroyed his arse with firepower before shooting him through the back a couple of times as well.

And just as this happened, the entire roof came off the building. There was a blinding white light everywhere and, as I suddenly remembered hearing on a late night Radio 4 theological programme about how the real date for the millennium was 3 pm on December 5th 1999, I felt myself being transported upwards, up and into the ether. And the only thing that I could think of was, shit, I forgot to drink the whiskey. I bet that there are no hangovers in heaven.

IGNORE RUTH KETTLE'S LIES!

TIM TELSA

6/2/99.

I bought this diary today. I intend this book to be a dialogue of my political activities, thoughts and things that take place, which may or may not in the future be of interest to the following of the political issues that I personally set up.

As said in my last diary, the Alconbury Nine left an important message to the left, and that was to be wary of the legal implications of keeping a diary. However, in this context, I believe that the work I have done in fighting for revolution is both important in the name of that revolution itself, and in the name of guerrilla cease-fire in Northern Ireland. The 'Guerilla Press' are guerrillas, and this diary is intended, ultimately, as a manual in guerrilla warfare. So, with that opening, I open up the first entry for the current day.

Today was a particularly important day, as it was today that I finally confessed to the Chaplain: not only to Strangeways and the bombing of 10 Downing Street, but also to upholding the assignment I was given to crucify Jesus Christ. I explained that the crucifixion was very probably an assignment given by the I.R.A. in response to the previous actions mentioned; those being the two acts perpetrated deliberately to instigate negotiations with Irish paramilitaries, negotiations that initiated the cease-fire. Even so, it was still the fault of myself that Jesus was killed, and I have to take responsibility for that. Chaplain seemed to understand, but she didn't give me advice. I will go to church tomorrow, to see if anything changes.

Received a letter from the Labour Party this morning, asking me to fill out a form allowing my bank to credit them money on a monthly basis. Intend to send it back to them with a letter explaining that I can't afford to if the Welfare State will insist on paying hospital patients the pittance of £12.50 per week. They seem to be able to justify keeping people locked up in places like this, unable to work or vote, screwed up on forced injections and crowded together, giving us no money at all. Maybe one day I'll get my say at the negotiating table, and demand a living wage from the Welfare State.

It would appear that the left have boycotted my mail. I still receive mail, but the vast majority of the letters I send still elicit no reply. Despite this, the Guerilla Press will continue whatever. More letters tonight.

7/2/99.

Sundays in this psychiatric hospital are very boring indeed. I feel compelled to write about the incidents of last night, today being a day uneventful and boring.

Marylin phoned last night, about half past nine. She was on the phone for about an hour, ranting. She seems able to talk non-stop: she could go on forever. Whilst on the phone, I was handed the day's mail, which I opened as I was on the phone.

Yesterday's mail was basically bad news. The first letter I opened was from a medical charity writing to me in order to ask for a donation (they wanted £250). Not being able to make a donation of that sort of money, I told Marylin, who asked me to forward it to her: she wants to raise some funds for them. I forwarded it onto her this morning, also posting mail to Adam and Hawkzine concerning the fanzine I posted last week.

This piece of mail was OK. I think they must have got my address through the Labour Party. However, the rest of my mail was more disappointing.

The first of these letters was from Griffin Book Distribution, returning a letter with a slip attached, impolitely demanding: "Please take us off your distribution list." This I have happily done. The next letter was from the Broadcasting Standards Complaints Commission, stating, in official terms, that they wouldn't be able to help my case, due to my being unable to prove that any particular programme was reporting me specifically. I have kept the letter, so that I can write to them again when I get a personal slander that I can quote.

I didn't go to church today, I felt too tired. However, it may be that yesterday's claim to be responsible for the I.R.A. cease-fire may be able to help me. I wait to see what happens.

This week I am reading a book of essays by Aleister Crowley. Although it doesn't go into details about the practice of magick, it is well written, but at the same time I'm not really inspired by it. I am trying to take it as an exercise in "true will" to read it before next Saturday, when I can go into Cambridge where I intend to buy some books on the Enochian system of magick. I am still cursing my stamps with the blood sacrifice of a pin, although, at present, there is no longer an active Guerilla Press or C.C.A.

8/2/99.

Went to maths today. Very boring, but I think it might come in useful. I have been budgeting my money to be able to buy a mobile phone so that I can set up on the internet. This will be on the condition that the hospital allow me to do so, or otherwise the money will allow me to print another pamphlet. The thing is, now that I have cut down my smoking, intending to stop, I now think about spending my money on other things. I am trying to stop completely, but as it stands I have cut down.

No mail today, but on the subject of money, I have applied to the Princes Youth Trust for a grant to set up a radical bookshop on the internet (Radical BookSite). I have also written to granny to ask her to help me out with the phone charges. I think she will, although I'm not so sure about getting a loan from the Princes Trust.

Myself and Janet (my friend from the other Bungalow) are both having trouble with people not responding to our mail. With Janet it upsets her if she doesn't get any response to her mail. With me, I am actually trying to benefit the cause of the revolution, and nothing is happening with it. I need a response to the Radical Presses Register idea - and if nothing is happening with the idea, then what am I supposed to do? Marylin (my pen-pal) confirms my idea when she says it is a definite possibility that my post is being boycotted. It could be. But if it is, then why?

Went to see an exhibition of art at the local Community Art Centre today. This was a collection of photo-collages that we had put together ourselves in an art session. One of these photos was of myself wearing my Astronauts T-shirt with my head missing from the photo. I took the opportunity of being the Avant Bard, by going along in the same Astronauts T-shirt. I got a funny reaction!

Still planning to go home to see Mum in a couple of weeks' time. She has found some anarchist literature for me: stuff that she found in a car boot sale. The stuff she sent already looks really interesting, although I haven't had the chance to read it yet. Working on an anthology of blue drugs from a medical index that I found on a skip. Calling it "Campaign Against Blue Smarties" with a pseudo-Nazi line, taking the piss. I'm thinking about printing it if the hospital don't let me set up with a modem. Sitting here in front of the T.V., desperate for another cigarette. More news tomorrow.

9/2/99.

Nothing really exciting in the post toady; a mailout from someone calling themselves the 'United Nations Association Trust', and an internal letter from Advocacy. The letter from the UNA Trust was about refugees, and I would like to send them some money, but I can't afford to. The letter from Advocacy was about how patients feel Advocacy works, they are going to send someone around with a questionnaire on the 16th. Still no feedback from the Radical Presses Register mailout. I wonder what's going on?

Put some money in the bank earlier. This morning was my first opportunity to use my unescorted pass. As somebody who has actually helped the 'peace process' in Northern Ireland so directly, I am treated very badly by the State (considering most other political prisoners have been released from jail). I feel tempted to contact the UNA Trust about seeking asylum myself. The problem is that I don't think they'd believe my case. Amnesty International didn't.

At the moment I am saving up to get myself connected to the internet. There are advantages with having got myself in mental hospital instead of prison. One of them is that I can keep running the Guerilla Press. That means that the next step is setting up on the net, although it may be the case that the staff won't let me. Should this be the case, the money will go into printing the plans for the Vectron rocket, and distributing them to the left. These blueprints will be published in the form of a pamphlet, and I will send it out free to the anarchists again; although I will include a copy of my own leaflet with the mailout at the same time. I still doubt that I will actually be able to sell any, but the dissemination of propaganda is the most important issue. The idea of putting a rocket in the sky is revolutionary in its own way; Pirate Radio rockets may be the future.

The principle of the Zodiac Rocket, as I call it, could easily be used as a missile design, although I would prefer it not to be used for that purpose. The plans will explain the idea further when they are published, although, as said, this will only come about as a result of the hospital not allowing me to set up on the net. The principle, in short, is that of magnetic coils working on opposite polarities, but I'll explain that later. It's just that it occurs to me that, if this invention were used as a missile, there could be a humorous reaction from the State (HA HA).

10/2/99.

It has occurred to me that the M.M.R. will cost too much to patent. The situation is that I have distributed the rough plans to the A.A.A. and, now that it has come to me that I just don't have the money to patent the idea, it is only now a matter of time before the project gets into the hands of counter-terrorist factions in order to threaten my cease-fire. Therefore I am resorting to blackmail.

The plan is to raise the necessary funds to be able to print the blueprints as a political sequel to *How to Make a Petrol Bomb*, send something like 500 copies to someone like the A.L.F. support group, and then to threaten a bank or someone to pay a "sum of cash" in order for the plans not to be distributed. It still strikes me as being amusing, that the military could find themselves under fire from a completely new form of rocket technology.

Saw a psychiatrist from a hospital in London this morning. She seemed quite nice, but asked a lot of questions. It looks like I might get moved out some time before July. If this is the case, I can use my time to work on my M.M.R. prototype from my Dad's workshop address. It will be another step towards my freedom, and I intend to use my time getting into politics; possibly organising more riots with the AKSMOS flag, or possibly making speeches. Either way, the plan now is to keep my nose clean until I move out, and then to go underground in the squat scene to organise Pirate Radio.

The rocket idea could eventually be used to put a Pirate Radio relay into sub-orbital space, and this is something that I could get into building after discharge. People at the workshop have told me that they'll help me get such a project "off the ground," as the Mars Project joke went. If this is to be possible, then I will have to employ the expertise of my younger brother, who is doing a diploma in electronics. I find it difficult to describe the actual technology necessary to build a satellite myself. There are a lot of things I could do when I get discharged, but the plan for the time being is to keep my nose clean and not to blow my front.

No mail came for me today. Again no mail: this must surely prove the apathy, or possibly the small-mindedness of the left. The current next step with the postal campaign is to either distribute or try to sell the plans for the M.M.R. I am still expecting a book through the post on Computer Hacking. Once that gets here, assuming it ever does, then I may be able to write some sort of dialogue on hacking before the end of the year. But it aggravates me that the people I write to will persistently refuse to reply to my mail. From A.C.F. to the A.L.F., there seems to be a deliberate lack of response. Is it because I am a psychiatric patient I wonder?

11/2/99.

Whilst watching Channel Four last night, I saw an advert with a freephone number advertising a free "inventors pack." I phoned the number, and eventually got through to a very rushed telephone woman on the other end, who took my address and phone number. Before putting the phone down, I had time to explain something about the M.M.R. idea.

I explained, in the short time that I had, that I had invented a satellite communications rocket, and that I had already received the documentation that the application for the patent had been registered. I also explained that I could not afford to pursue the patent, and that I had already distributed the plans to the A.A.A. (an anarchist group). I went on to explain that, if I did not get my patent registered within the allotted period, then it was only a matter of time before the plans got into the hands of the I.R.A. (an Irish Nationalist terrorist organisation). The woman on the end of the phone told me to get a pen.

When I had got back with the pen, the phone had been put down, so I tried again. Eventually, after some negotiation, another woman gave me the phone number for a group in Dublin who could possibly give me a grant. So I phoned the number this morning, but was unable to get through. So the plan stays as it was in the first place.

Received a lot of post through the hospital bureaucracy this morning. Marylin wrote a letter. For some reason she seems upset that I printed the leaflet concerning the 'Freepost' idea. I cannot understand why, but she has now gone and contacted her solicitor about it, as well as getting in touch with mine. If I understood what had upset her, then I'd apologise, but I don't know how I've upset her in the first place! This could get me in trouble with the hospital again, and that could mean anything from a deferral of my discharge, to a referral to Rampton ('Special Hospital'). She's also pissed me off by telling me I did the wrong thing getting myself sectioned. She says that it means I'm not a political prisoner. I suppose that just about sums up the attitude of the left towards the Guerilla Press.

Received another letter this morning from the Revolutionary Socialist Network. Sent me a copy of 'Heresy', their magazine. Looks interesting, although I have only just browsed through it. Sent some hunger strike leaflets and an R.P.R. leaflet in return. Still no feedback about the Radical Presses Register. I wait.

12/2/99.

Nothing of note has happened in the hospital today, although this is the normal thing. I have been writing manically over the past few days, and this has drained me. Despite having nothing to mention, I received some mail this morning.

The first thing to note, is that I was sent a copy of South Cambridgeshire Labour Party newsletter. I have not read it, and I intend not to reply. The mass boycott of our mail was organised by the press under the regime of the Labour Party, and therefore I refuse to reply to them. They wrote to me yesterday to tell me that my bank account wouldn't allow them to take out a direct debit. They're the government for God's sake! Why do they need permission from me to take money?

Hawkzine sent me a postcard this morning. The bloke who runs it isn't very good at English, so it was difficult to decipher what he was saying. The gist of it says that he has a problem with lots of leaflets being sent through the post, although he did agree to send out the leaflets I sent him, so I wrote back to say thank you. Also received two copies of SchNEWS, neither of which I have yet read, although I intend to read them either tonight or tomorrow morning.

Wrote to Marylin earlier, basically to ask what had I done to offend her? If I haven't yet documented it, she seems to have been offended by a leaflet I photocopied, trying to subvert for the purposes of the postage stamps boycott that she was organising. The idea was essentially to put 'Freepost Guevara RM18' on the top of the envelope, the normal address and an 'if undelivered' address on the back. She asked me to distribute the idea to as many different people as possible, so I produced a leaflet. Now she wants to take me to court!

If she does take me to court, I don't believe she has a legal leg to stand on. The thing is that now she's getting offensive about my being locked up in a mental hospital: "not a political prisoner!" I have written to her telling her that I am: it is a conspiracy of the State and their press that is keeping me here, and I am running a public pressure campaign to shed light upon the media monitoring of thought.

Anyway, nothing else has happened today, except for the writing I have been doing for these two Volumes of work. The deadline is the end of the year, after which I will be absconding to hand myself in with a leaflet offering to sell my story to the press. Although I am now in a psychiatric hospital, I have been on the run for the past ten years, and I laugh every day. I have engineered this situation and I am not mad. I am a weird Satanic Penguin of the Narley!

13/2/99.

Spoke to Dad today whilst in Royston. The conversation was about setting up on the internet. I do not have his approval, and granny says she is unwilling to pay the phone bill for the project. It now looks like I will have to wait until I get discharged before I can set up.

Aside from that, things are going all right. Although I had no mail through my Dad's address, things are still moving. I am writing to a number of Catholic "directors of communication" that I photocopied at the library, sending them a chain letter. I am pissed off that I wasn't represented by the Labour Party's "Good Friday" agreements, when it was directly my own activities that led to them. The letter will explain this, saying that it was Strangeways that threatened the State to step down to the I.R.A., and the bombing of Downing Street that forced the government to surrender to guerrillas. This, as well as the assassination of Jesus possibly being the signal for the I.R.A. cease fire. I believe I have a right to issue the C.C.A. demands.

The plan is, therefore, to write a duplicate letter to twenty contacts, explaining this from the C.C.A. as the front organisation for AKSMOS, the prostitutes' guerrilla. I plan to threaten, through the C.C.A., that AKSMOS intend to resume activities on the 19th of June 2000. That gives me just enough time to send a number of letter bombs before I hand myself in with a leaflet at Stonehenge for the New Age.

On to the next bit, it occurs to me that if I can't set up on the internet before June next year, and it might not be practical for me to do so, then it is possible to print the designs for the M.M.R. much sooner than I had originally thought. Therefore I intend to take the originals to the printers next Tuesday at the latest. It is a bit of a problem that I can't set up on the internet beforehand, but it's like that and that's the way it is. Plans for distribution etc. will be discussed as they become apparent, but I don't really expect much of a response.

What I'm thinking of is asking the A.L.F. to keep about 200 copies, and writing a blackmail demand to force the government into considering our demands under Stormont, having the blueprints to fall back on if it goes wrong. The intention is to wait for the A.L.F. support group to reply, before writing to them to ask them if they can keep the prints, and then distribute them in the event of my writing a letter from prison. Have to make a mental note that the blurb is going to have to be fairly inflammatory if it is going to work. That won't be too difficult though.

14/2/99.

Due to a trip to the pub earlier today, I have done very little work. However, I did tidy up my room and write the chain letter to 'Directors of Communication' for the Catholic church.

The letter turned out to be shorter than I had expected because I was drunk. Even so, it carried the main points and the general gist. Points made were, in short:

a) That the C.C.A. are the spokesperson organisation for AKSMOS.

b) That AKSMOS were responsible for the bombing of Downing Street and Strangeways.

c) That with these points taken into account, AKSMOS were responsible for both I.R.A. cease-fire, and the Stormont negotiations combined.

In this we have reissued the three demands, making it clear to the Church that the B.B.C. etc. are using black magick to monitor thought, and that this must end. The letter concludes that, if demands are not met, then AKSMOS will resume operations in Summer 2000.

The letters have not yet been sent, although they are now all in their envelopes with an R.P.R. leaflet. I have sent them through the 'Freepost Guevara' scheme, enclosing another leaflet explaining the idea. As there were a few copies of the main letter left, I sent them to the I.W.W., also through the 'Freepost Guevara' scheme.

This just about concludes this dialogue of guerrilla activity for today, although I should write an account of St. Valentine's day. Sent a letter to Janet on Friday: a St. Valentine's 'anti-card.' Also sent her a number of leaflets, marking the envelope 'Strictly Confidential'. The staff passed strict rules last year, that I was not allowed to send or distribute work of any kind at all to the patients of the hospital; apparently because it could be considered 'subversive'. Therefore, if anything gets sent through the Guerilla Press, it goes in complete secrecy. I now have a 'post box pass', allowing me to walk down to the post box with a member of staff, if I can arrange it. I plan to exploit this tomorrow, with the letters to the church. Anyway, back to the point. This is the sort of draconian control ethic that exists in hospital, that has always been used against me and my work. It was only last year that the 'Statement ov Intent' was confiscated from the local bookshop, as only one example of the oppression of my work. Therefore I write this second volume, as a conclusion to the work of the C.C.A., taking advantage of this as my last piece of writing before losing the relative freedom that I currently enjoy.

Tomorrow I will write another letter to the A.L.F., to try to get them in correspondence over the M.M.R. project. Let's see how it goes.

15/2/99.

Letter from the British Library: 'Thank you for the leaflet about the Radical Presses Register. The advantage of I.S.B.N.s for libraries is that they are unique to a specific title or edition of a title and thus make it easier to identify material, e.g. to order it or to meet a reader's enquiry. I enclose details of British Library programmes which I hope will be of interest.'

Some interest from the British Library about the R.P.R. scheme. I received a letter this morning from them, enclosing a number of leaflets about them and what they do. This is the first letter of interest about the R.P.R. and it is welcome.

What the British Library are saying, is that they prefer the idea of the old I.S.B.N. system, as it makes it easier for librarians to find specific books under specific categories etc. which is something I should have paid more thought to. There probably won't be much time before setting up the R.P.R. and handing myself in, because I won't have access to the internet before I am discharged. Even with this, it only leaves me a year before I hand myself in to the police for riot offences. Even so, for the purposes of documentation, I will have to remember the following points:

a) That I will have to have a table of book categories on the internet page, that can link to individual books.

b) I will have to put publishers' addresses next to the book titles as often as possible, and be able to sell books through the programme as well, and:

c) I will have to inform the British Library first of all books registered under the scheme.

Although I will probably not be able to run the project for very long, I will probably be able to get someone to take the idea over for me. As well as which, I document the idea within these pages, as an example of the value of the printed word in guerrilla struggle.

I also wrote to A.K. Distribution today, concerning the book I ordered from them last month. I have heard nothing from them, and I am worried that I might be getting ripped off. There is an old motto that says: 'If you live outside the law, you have to be honest'. The R.P.R. will have strict rules not to rip anyone off on book orders. If we are to do something productive, we will have to earn a reputation.

Took advantage of my first 'post box pass' today. With another two escorted trips to the post box, I will be able to go there as often as I like. Posted those letters to the church this morning, and I am wondering if I will get a response. Still waiting to send letters to A.K., the British Library and Black Flag etc. Still haven't written to the A.L.F. support group, but I'll do that later today or early tomorrow.

16/2/99.

For the next few days, I will have to get on with my psychology coursework. I will have until March 1st to complete my first piece of coursework, and to do another two. But I feel confident that I can do it if I get on to it now.

It has been a productive day for the M.M.R. project. I wrote that letter to the A.L.F., asking if they'd like to stash, say, 500 copies of the printed plans for the rocket. But another thing happened today.

The post didn't arrive until two o'clock, but when it eventually did arrive, there was a letter from a group in Ireland, something to do with inventions. This group, who I believe to be genuine, say they are some sort of service for people to get their ideas patented. They sent a form, which I filled out, to do with the rough idea for the invention. I think they are some sort of company to help inventors get their ideas patented, provided they can pay for it.

Therefore I had to write to them, explaining that I am trying to get the idea patented, but that I can't afford it. So, what I am hoping for, is that these people will be able to put the money up front to help me patent the rocket. Failing that, I have planned to distribute the idea to anarchists around the world, as described earlier. The plan, however, was that I was going to do that anyway.

What I intend to do, is to wait until my idea has been patented, assuming that I can do that, and then to circulate the idea on a wide scale through printing the idea as a pamphlet.

Interesting situation in London today. Four hundred protesters stormed the Turkish Embassy, apparently in response to the leader of the P.K.K. group having been arrested, I think in Turkey. A good protest organised on an international scale, it has support from the C.C.A., although without funds the Guerilla Press cannot actively support, however much we would like to. However, I would like to document one point, and that is that I find it quite serious that these protesters are actually threatening to **set themselves on fire**. This I must disagree with, as we need to keep as many good protesters as we possibly can. Although the Guerilla Press support direct action, **we cannot support people setting themselves on fire**. Victims of arson are the political victims of the continuation of the revolution: threatening to set themselves on fire is taking the situation too far. However, in saying that, it is not for me to dispute the actions of those involved in holy war. It is just that I would like to see protest without victims of fire.

17/2/99.

The siege of the British Embassy by this country's Turkish population continues, with an undisclosed number of P.K.K. members actually occupying the embassy, declaring that they are on hunger strike: "until death." This protest continues on an international scale, with riots and a report of one fifteen year old girl actually setting herself on fire. I.T.N. reports claimed to 'examine' how this could happen on a world-wide scale, concluding only that they had their own T.V. channel. I would like to offer more support, but I don't know how to, and anyway, this project is more important, if that can be said.

Completed my first piece of coursework for my psychology course today, and I hope to complete the second, which I have now started, and put them both in the post tomorrow. The second piece of coursework is based on an observation study, which I did today, standing at the Pelican Crossing in Royston for ten minutes.

Little post today, except for a response to my mail from the Princes Trust. This concerns the R.P.R. project to set up an alternative system of book numbering, eventually in order to set up a radical bookshop on the internet. Although I will not actually be able to properly set this up if I am to hand myself in for the Summer Solstice 2000, the Princes Trust seem to be saying that I might be entitled to a grant, and I intend to pursue this idea in order to document the idea in this diary: firstly to help others who may be inspired by the R.P.R. idea to set up projects of their own, but also to screw some money out of the State and then document myself doing it for the use of further correspondence with those I consider to be the revolutionaries of the future.

The Princes Trust seem to be offering grants to people who have been unemployed for a while (in my case all my life), and then who are "disadvantaged" (in my case wrongly diagnosed with paranoid schizophrenia). All the same, however just this scheme may first come across as, it is nothing more than a justification for this country's bastard capitalist dictatorship. Further than that, it is a front for the sick monarchist, Prince Charles. I intend to take every opportunity to expose this con, to rip it off and take advantage of it as I hand myself in.

18/2/99.

Book 1, *Collected Essays*, was near completion today when I printed out 'Theft' one more time, and already Ruth Kettle has threatened to take complete responsibility for the whole project, by saying that it was her 'who wrote it'. She is fascist scum, and I have no qualms about slandering her, as she would amount to libel if I had respect enough from nurses and the law to take her to court for it. For the individual who publicly declared cease-fire in the I.R.A., they have some nerve, the way they treat me. I have threatened letter bombs to resume activities on the 19/6/00. That will change her.

Kurdish demonstrators occupying the Greek Embassy in London gave themselves up today, at about 3.00 pm; and the implications for world-wide revolution are only just beginning to be discussed, or considered, by the press. I can only say that I support the issue, although now the plan is to hand myself in, and as I am already in psychiatric hospital, there is little I can do to support it. Even so, our reporting has helped their case (this 'reporting' being in the context of the media reporting what I think).

Completed my application to the Princes Trust today, walked down to the post box and, being someone who has always fought for revolution, do you really think I would conform to this capitalist front for the monarchy shit? Here's the plan.

I intend to carry on with the R.P.R. project, getting a grant to set up on the internet. I intend to exploit this opportunity to sell books on shoplifting etc., including my own work, and then do a runner with the remaining funds, and to use these funds to print both volumes of *Chaoticism*. Once printed, these books will legally stand as my confession to Strangeways and terrorist offences linked to the Guerilla Press, and I will be spending the rest of my life in prison. But this in the cause of the revolution, is far more important than being the advocate of revolution that I once was.

Back on to the subject of Book 1: I am pleased with it, and I feel that it is well worth the Guerilla label. I am trying to get the pages numbered before tomorrow afternoon, when I will try to get a trip into Royston, in order to take it to the printers for three photocopies. I am now getting towards the end of my role as an active revolutionary guerrilla. I no longer feel in touch with the grass roots movement of the revolution, and I am getting ready for the rest of my life in prison. As I write this diary, I am setting up for this, and once I have finished it, I will be selling the story to the papers in order to print it. This is what I intend to leave to the revolution, the world I could have made, and Beelzebub, whom I loved, but never knew.

19/2/99.

Writing prematurely, on Thursday night, it occurs to me that I have not made my point about Strangeways and the I.R.A. cease-fire, and the subject now should be to concentrate on how I am going to get these Volumes published. I plan to rip off the Princes Trust; failing that I could try to do a press release to try and sell my story. This Volume doesn't need to be published yet: I will be able to sell this diary at a later stage, if necessary selling it to the papers. And so this diary now documents 'The Conspiracy of the Guerilla Press.'

Volume 1 is now complete (again), but what strikes me is that, in its own context, the words 'anarchist' and 'fascist' could be used interchangeably. Now starts the process of trying to get the book published. As a documentation of the C.C.A. transition from some sort of feminism, to an extreme form of chauvinism, I could think about selling it to right-wing publishers. Even so, I am unlikely to sell it to a publisher, so the plan is still to publish it through ripping off the Princes Trust. This being Volume 2, it will serve as evidence in court as 'conspiracy to defraud', as well as being a confession to Strangeways and the bombing of Downing Street,. but I will already be on my way to prison for defrauding the monarchy in the first place, and the plan was to hand myself in anyway.

Today's entry is short, as I have a screaming headache. Just to mention that I didn't get into Royston, the book didn't come through the post, and neither did the funds from Dad. I visit Mum in Swansea tomorrow.

5.30 pm: My headache has now gone. Janet received a pile of newsletters and other stuff from the Movement Against the Monarchy this morning. This gets to me, as I distributed 100 copies of a leaflet with their address at the bottom of it, and have received no response from them myself. What gets to me, is that no one has told me why I am getting such a lack of response to my mail. Have I been boycotted, or what?

Book 1 finished this morning, and it occurs to me that my politics are very extreme, and may not actually be right. I seem to have invented Sadism as a political issue.

Is this why I get no response to my mail?
Continuing with my book on Aleister Crowley.

20/2/99.

Last night was nearly my second fun trip back to the Secure Ward. I phoned Mum, to tell her that the train was getting in at ten past two, which it did, and then happened to mention that I was reading Crowley, which she disagrees with. Ten minutes later I phoned her back, basically saying that I wouldn't be coming if she wasn't going to respect my religious principles. Soon afterwards I was on the verge of a near-relapse, feeling guilty about what I had just done.

As it goes, I did get back to Swansea for the weekend, and it is really nice to be here. I was using Abra Melin last night for all books to come to me, and it seems to be materialising already. I was reading *The Mars Mystery* on the train down here, and when I got here, I found three books waiting for me. These were:

a) *Act for Yourselves*, by Kropotkin,

b) *How We Shall Bring About the Revolution*, by Emile Patuad and Emile Pouget, and:

c) *Freedom to Roam*, by Harold Scunthorpe.

This, on top of the books I received from Manor Books, seems to be a lot more than just a coincidence. I plan to further my knowledge of ritual magick, and get into using Abra Melin properly for the Guerilla Press. Tonight's entry stops short, due to nothing political having taken place; a long day travelling to Wales.

21/2/99.

The concept of doing a runner with a grant from the Princes Trust is now beginning to become a dilemma. It's just the concept of being arrested before everything is finalised. I suppose that just by writing this book, I am putting my neck on the line, and I will have to go into hiding if I print it rather than handing myself in. But then again, I don't have to publish this book, and setting up in business, if it happens, could provide the income to print books 1 and 2. Doing a runner with the money may not seem like such a good idea after all.

At the same time, I cannot stay on the run forever, and the concept of leaving these Volumes to the revolutionaries of the future may be more important. Therefore I believe that it may be the answer to many problems to publish these works anonymously. There seems no point in printing more and more Volumes that'll never be published, and the idea of getting someone to publish them for me seems like a much better idea. Still, I feel it important that my work be published, for the benefit of the history books if nothing else.

As regards the sacred magick of Abra Melin the Mage: I acquired another book this morning, a book on the conspiracy of alien landings on the planet Earth. That, as well as the book I am currently reading (*The Mars Mystery*, by Graham Hancock), should leave me with a view.

I write this entry on the train getting back from Swansea. I had a home visit, but I have started planning my escape. I intend to change my name by deed poll, and learn to speak German before eventually escaping to Germany.

Intending to speak to the hospital vicar again on Monday, basically to ask where I stand on the issue of the I.R.A. cease-fire and the crucifixion. All being well, I will ask her to help me to abscond. The only thing stopping me from absconding today is that I have to stay around for my psychology exam in June. Concerning that, the next three days are going to be entirely taken up with doing my coursework; it has to be done by March the First.

Hoping to receive some cash in the post when I arrive back. This will pay for the photocopying of Book 1. I need three copies. As well as that, I expect *Mein Kampf* to have come into the bookshop in Royston on Tuesday.

Nothing else of real importance to write today. Trip home held up movements since Friday. More tomorrow.

22/2/99.

Fate plays some funny games. Just as I have decided to do a runner to Germany and rip off the Princes Trust, things start taking place.

At about half past two this afternoon, I received a phone call from an American bloke, claiming to be from the I.T.E. (Information Technology Exchange - the people who were originally interested in the M.M.R.) This bloke, and I can't remember his name, was saying that he had received the plans to the Rocket Ship, and asked to make arrangements to phone me up tomorrow with "some more questions." I told him that I'd be around tomorrow at about one o'clock. The A.L.F. have not written back to me; so this may be productive.

After that had taken place, I phoned a publisher: 'Chatto & Windus' in London. After some negotiation, they eventually expressed a real interest in reading Book 1. So I photocopy it, hopefully tomorrow, weigh it and post it, hopefully on Wednesday.

That's about it as regards the Guerilla Press today. I received no mail, but I would like to write a note about Abra Melin the Mage. I have been practising a lot of magick over the last few days. The most interesting of these spells is that I have drawn a number of Talismans, with a sigil for conjuration on one side of the paper, and a sigil for love on the other. I am doing this so that Beelzebub will once more return to me in evil reincarnated as beauty. One of these Talismans I burned; the other I hid in the back of the Malleus Malificarum with my crucifix. Now just to wait, although I have received no books today.

I did my coursework for psychology earlier. I had five subjects doing a simple memory experiment. It went quite well, although four out of five of them remembered nearly all of the words, which surprised me. So I wrote it up earlier, and sent it through the post shortly afterwards. It should get there in time. That leaves me with only one piece of coursework left to do, which I will do tomorrow.

Now that I have just about finished psychology, I will be studying on quite a high level. I would like to start a diploma in political study as a mature student in London. I am looking forward to being discharged, and when that happens, the only thing that can stop me is being sectioned again. This is where I prove the world wrong. I make one step after another: only small, and not for mankind, but for the future and for me!

23/2/99.

It now seems obvious that the idea for the Radical Presses Register isn't going to come together. At the same time, ideas of doing a runner are also looking as if they are not going to happen. Nobody seems to be really interested in the R.P.R., although I have interest from the British Library, and I hope for a grant from the Princes Trust, and if I get it I will use it for the project, rather than ripping them off.

My plan so far has been to sit tight, staying on the run for Strangeways, but playing the game as far as I am capable. The plan is to wait until I get arrested, and then sell my story to the papers via my solicitor; sending the manuscript to Volume 1, and using the money to publish it myself in prison. That is assuming that I can't get anyone else to publish it before that.

But whilst on the subject of the first Volume, I seem to have some interest from a publisher. Because of this, I have taken the manuscript to the printers today for three copies. I have also bought three files, and I hope to have two manuscripts in the post next week. All in all, this has taken up almost all of the revolutionary funds. Sending them will cost more. But if it works in the name of the revolution, then it has to be worthwhile.

On to the subject of the M.M.R. The American bloke phoned back this afternoon, interrupting me having lunch with Janet. He asked me a couple of questions: in particular he asked whether I'd mind the Rocket being built from recycled materials. Then he said that I'd still have to pay for the idea myself, which I won't be able to unless I get the book published. He said he'd phone back tomorrow.

The resistance of the Kurds in London and around the world is now over, leaving the press to wonder what happened, and the left to wonder how. Although the situation has now been swept under the carpet, seemingly by all, it was significant, and it led the Guerilla Press to ask a lot of questions about how our politics related to it. But what is important, is that world-wide demonstrations by the Kurds were influenced by, and in support of, a guerrilla leader. Therefore we should not underestimate our role in revolution. Prostitutes earning respect in society through taking up arms would have to be supported by riots: and we have declared our support for the P.K.K.

24/2/99.

No mail came today, and this has annoyed me as I am trying to give up smoking. Finished reading that book on Mars, and started reading *Alien Base* by Timothy Good. Still my book on computer hacking hasn't come through the post, and I am beginning to think that I may have been ripped off. I await a response from the Princes Youth Trust.

Received another phone call this morning from the I.T.E., who seem to be interested in the M.M.R. They've spoken about a loan and, as the A.L.F. seem to be not in the least bit interested, then this might be the way to go. It seems to be the only thing that is going right at the moment.

At the present point I am thinking of printing a pamphlet on U.F.O.s for the Guerilla Press; photocopying say 100 copies, as with *Thirteen*. This would be a change from the strategy of the Guerilla Press so far, and may serve to be useful in the name of selling more books. There may be a bigger audience for books on U.F.O.s, and I might be able to start selling stuff in alternative bookshops. If I can stop smoking then I may well be able to afford it.

That said, the main issue of the Guerilla Press is in trying to sell *Chaoticism*. I took the manuscript to the printers yesterday afternoon, expecting to have a trip into Royston today, asking for three photocopies. The downside is that this will take most of the revolutionary funds. I have bought three files and two parcel boxes. So I intend to send the manuscripts next Tuesday - one to Chatto & Windus, who have expressed an interest in my work, and one to my solicitor to look after. In the event of my being arrested at any point I intend to sell my story to the News of the World, spending the money on publishing Volume 1 privately. In the happier event of my not being arrested, I still intend to raise the relevant funds, hopefully through setting up the R.P.R., in order to publish it that way.

But it really rests on my giving up smoking. So far it is going quite well. I have given up twice before, and I think I can do it again. What it means is that I will be answerable to no one; I will be free financially to do as I please. I will be healthier. I will have more money to spend on books. And if I can sell my invention, then everything's sorted. I will be on the path to set up publishing, and that's the future I want.

Finished the last piece of coursework for my psychology course yesterday. Now I just have to wait for the exam before I can hopefully get into University. I applied for a prospectus last night. Not bad for someone who left school with no qualifications and a drug problem.

25/2/99.

Today I am not in the best of moods, as I am trying to stop smoking. Nothing came for me in the post today, which makes me more grumpy. I am beginning to think that I have been ripped off by A.K. Books, and I don't know what to do. To make things worse, I dropped my dinner all over the floor this evening, breaking the pie dish and losing most of the rest of my food.

The rest of the day hasn't been so bad, however. Sadly no shopping trip happened today, so I intend to go shopping tomorrow, if the staff allow me to. I have to pick up my photocopying, and I am hoping that my books will have come into the shop by tomorrow.

As for the Guerilla Press, we still continue. There was a session over the flats this afternoon, discussing the project that could be set up for the hospital by the local arts co-operative. After a long discussion, I came up with the idea of possibly putting together a compilation of patients' poetry, and printing it as a project for the hospital. If this happened it would employ people's talents and interests: it would involve the interest in writing poetry that most of the group have, it would involve someone's interest in photography, it would involve my own interest in mail art and printing, and it would involve drama in the context of doing a press release for the book. I would like this to come together, as it would be a project for the Guerilla Press, and above all else it would be fun in the context of everyone pulling their interests together to do something.

I met the vicar today, passing through the main building. I've arranged a meeting on Saturday, and I will have a couple of issues to discuss. The first of these is, if the crucifixion was the reason for I.R.A. cease-fire, then where do I stand with the Catholic church? The second of these is, will the church help me abscond? I need to be in a place with access to the internet so that I can continue the R.P.R.

Still not much feedback about the R.P.R., although I have applied for this grant from the Princes Trust which, if it comes, could help me set up. I remind myself that it is commercially viable as the front for 'Radical Booksite' on the net.

26/2/99.

A couple of things happened last night. The first is that I got my mail: a New Scientist and a statement of declaration from the GANDALF campaign. It was nice to hear that this test case had been won, and it was equally nice that they'd remembered me. The next thing that happened was that I phoned up A.K. Distribution. It looks as if they haven't ripped me off after all. Apparently the particular book I ordered is out of stock, but they said that they'd received my letter, and that they haven't cashed my cheque yet.

Today I went into Royston and picked up three copies of the manuscript to Book 1. Also I wrote to my solicitor, to tell her that I was about to send her a copy as soon as I could get into Royston with the money to send them. Sent a letter to Delectus Books, and wrote a covering letter to Chatto & Windus press.

The post that came this morning was from the I.T.E. again. They are offering me a full "market search" for the M.M.R. project, including the stuff with the Patent Office. Unfortunately I can't afford the money, so I'm hoping that they'll offer me some sort of a loan or something. Still no response from the A.L.F.

Whilst in Royston this morning, I went into the bookshop. Still no sign of my books, although he says they'll be in on Thursday next week. I'm still sceptical though. I've been waiting for this book to come in for about a year now. The bookshop owner has a nerve, I feel. First he goes and blatantly grasses me up to the hospital because of the "pornographic and anarchistic" content of the book I asked him to stock for me; next he takes a year to order *Mein Kampf*, which I need for research purposes. He needs his shop burned down.

Back on to the subject of the A.L.F.: their not writing back to me has finally done in my faith in campaigning. I have received no mail from the vast majority of the people I write to, without any explanation as to why they won't write back, and no chance of a tribunal. It's not just animal rights groups, it's anarchists, booksellers, distribution, everyone. It's just that no one seems to be writing back to my mail. It upsets me, because I have done nothing wrong. This might lead me to finally wrapping up the C.C.A., to get into writing again, and not to try to be a part of the campaigning left anymore. If someone would tell me what I'd done wrong, then I could do something about it, but they don't. My reason for being in this hospital was, in the first place, political offences, but if I get sectioned for it, then what's the point? I talk to the vicar tomorrow about absconding. There seems no other choice.

27/2/99.

A lot of mail came today, and I had a chat with the vicar. Today's events deserve a proper write up, so I've decided to do a more thorough report tomorrow. Bought my brother a birthday card today.

28/2/99.

Met with the vicar yesterday, in short to ask where I stand in terms of being a member of the church. She seemed very reasonable, saying that I would be welcome as a member of the congregation; so I intend to go to chapel later. I also asked her whether I should hand myself in, and whether I should abscond. To both of these questions, her answer was no, and I feel that I should take her advice.

Received a letter from Marylin last night. She seems to be very upset about the postage scam; she has gone as far as threatening to take me to court. She seems to think that I have hijacked her idea, and she has even written to my solicitor demanding an "out of court settlement" of £500! I wrote back to her last night, telling her straight that I couldn't afford it. Where am I supposed to get £500 from? I don't even know where the money for the M.M.R. project is coming from, let alone giving this nutcase sums of money like this. I really think that this has to be taken as another lesson in trusting people. No one is trustworthy.

More news from the anarchist scene. There is to be a day of protest against the 'G7' conference on June 18th, with an internationally co-ordinated protest being organised by a group somewhere in this country, although it isn't clear exactly where. All the same, their leaflet has an international contacts list, and I would like to get involved with this, although it may turn out to be difficult.

As well as this, I received another couple of leaflets from anarchist groups with information on a couple of conferences that are being organised, although I will not be able to attend these. Being the political prisoner of a mental hospital, my movements are restricted, and I intend to be held here until I start at University. This leaflet also advertised a number of publications, none of which I can afford.

I also received a few other letters - two letters about my coursework (psychology); a letter from the Legal Deposits Office, basically saying that they've received five copies of the leaflet I sent them (it is a legal requirement to send five copies of any publication to A.T. Smail); and an S.A.E. from someone in Yorkshire who is interested in 'The Cruxifyer' (that being the newssheet I was running whilst writing Book 2). But the most important letter I received yesterday was a leaflet from the anarchist bookshop in Brixton. It concerns an eviction.

This is quite important, as 121 Books has been a squatted bookshop for the past fifteen years. Now the council have eventually passed an eviction order on the place. Anyway, a fair few groups run from their address, so I have decided to offer a B.M. Box for them, so that they can continue to offer addresses for the various political groups that run from their address. I will write to them later to put the idea to them.

Anyway, I'll write replies today, and fill out my entry for the rest of the day tonight. Now I'll try to arrange a church trip.

3.30pm: Wrote replies to various people, and sent a stamped addressed envelope to a group called 'Escape' for a copy of their pamphlet. Also wrote to '121 Book Shop', offering to pay for a B.M. Box for them. There are a number of differing political groups that I know of operating from that address, and if I can afford to help them out, now that they face eviction, then I feel I will be doing my bit for anarchism.

Last night I sent a manuscript to one of my comrades in the S/M Pride scene. The manuscript was a short erotic piece that I wrote, and I have sent it to her in the hope that she might publish it. This is the same person who stopped writing to me in last year's diary, so I hope she will be writing back to me this time.

Apparently there is going to be bingo on tonight over at the Women's Bungalow. Nothing ever really happens in these places, so I feel I may take the opportunity to play - there's some stamps being given away as prizes. It just seems so typical of the situation I am in that the only thing going on is bingo! No pub trips, no takeaways. This on top of the fact that we have no social life outside these walls, that no one considers us political prisoners, and that we have no entitlement to work or vote.

Marylin has stirred the shit by demanding £500. I'd like to kill her. If it's not enough to be wrongly imprisoned, then this pisstaking of my poverty just goes too far. She's out.

1/3/99.

No post came today, and we have been told that if we want our mail, then we will have to wait until tomorrow. Not much has happened today, and I have taken a day off; cooking a meal for Janet.

Got the manuscripts in the post today, and it cost a lot less than I expected it to. That's one to the publisher, Chatto & Windus; and one copy to my solicitor, sent so that I have something to fall back on: paying for her to send it to a publishing printers in the event of my having to sell the story of how I organised Strangeways to the press. The positive side of that is, firstly, I have something to fall back on if I get arrested and secondly, that I don't have to worry about having a book published if I get sent to a 'special hospital'.

The plan for tomorrow is to write a supporters newsletter for the people on the contacts list. Marylin has been deleted from it. This is in order to keep the Guerilla Press active as a guerrilla front. Points that I intend to include are: the eviction of 121 Books and an appeal for funds to open a B.M. Box for them, as I have offered to do; Marylin and her insane demand for £500; the Vectron rocket (more recently the M.M.R.); and the June 18th 'Protest against Global Capitalism'. I intend to send one copy to everyone on the contacts list, with an editorial to the political groups who have written to me, and a copy of *Propaganda Groups* with a mention that it is for sale on orders of 100 or above. I should send a leaflet as well.

I still expect replies from the Princes Trust and the A.L.F. These are people who I expect to reply to my mail; the rest I don't expect replies from anymore. It wouldn't be unreasonable to expect replies, but they don't come. This problem is detailed more fully in Book 2, and I don't really have time to discuss it here. I should get on with completing Book 2 in the next few days.

As for not getting my mail delivered today, this just keeps happening. We have all been told that we will have to wait until tomorrow. I see this as a blatant violation of my human rights. It is a blatant escalation of being told that I am "obviously schizophrenic" because of the way I dress when I'm a traveller, and being told that I am "not capable of giving consent to medication," when I am the first psychiatric patient to complete a qualification in Psychology. It is an escalation of prejudice and persecution.

2/3/99.

A quiet but productive day. Something that I forgot to document yesterday is that I received another phone call from the I.T.E., asking about the M.M.R. project. Basically they are asking for nearly £400 to complete a "market search," including the cost of the patent. I can't afford this, so it's back to blackmailing the State. Still no response from the A.L.F.

Received a letter from my Granny this morning. Although I haven't yet replied, it was a nice letter, if what she said seemed ambiguous. She said I had been told where it stood with my phone bill by my Dad, but at the same time she said she was willing to pay my 'E-Mail costs'. This seems a bit strange; I'm not really sure what she was saying. I also received two copies of SchNEWS.

I did the first 'Guerilla Press SUPPORTERS NEWSLETTER' earlier. I have to say that I am pleased with the way it came out, it filled exactly one side of an A4 sheet. I included everything that was directly relevant, but then found that I had run out of envelopes. I now just have to wait until I can get into Royston to get some more. When I have done that I will send one to everyone on the contacts list. Phoned the printers earlier about another run of R.P.R. leaflets. I think it's worthwhile, although they will cost about £10 more than expected.

Again I find myself considering putting an advert in Peace News. This could be a good way of increasing the contacts list; at least it will be a good way of distributing more propaganda. It would also get my name around. Either way, I think it would be a worthwhile experiment. It's experimentation that makes a group worthwhile, and it seems like a good project. If all that I intend to do is to distribute more propaganda, then this has to be the way to do it.

The last project to write about today, is that I am planning to set up the R.P.R. with my own publication, 'Rules ov 'e". I intend to print this with my own money, if I can afford to, and give it the first R.P.R. cataloguing number. This will be sent to every 'Games Workshop' address, with a 'trade copy' cover, detailing the R.P.R. and a reduced trade price on the back. I will write a short scenario and include it in the rules as an example of how the game works. In the meantime I intend to play through the scenario and playtest the rules at the same time once I have written it. Then I will try selling it to the people who publish Role Playing Games, in the hope of it being accepted; in which case 1 will not have to print it myself.

It is my brother's birthday tomorrow, and I have sent him some money through the post. I hope it gets there tomorrow, as I don't know his current address. I have sent it to Mum to give to him. I am hoping it will have arrived and been forwarded to him by tomorrow.

3/3/99.

A bad day today. I didn't get into Royston. The injection hurt. Even so, I got some envelopes from a friend, and started the mailout for the Supporters Newsletter, although I don't expect a response. I think I'll have more to write tomorrow when I get back from Royston, assuming I manage to get there tomorrow.

4/3/99.

A better day today. No post came, although I did get into Royston. Went in before I had time to do my job, but I got most of what I needed. Took a copy of the R.P.R. leaflet to the printers - I've ordered a run of another 200 on purple paper. Whilst I was there I got six copies of the experimental map I have drawn for the Science Fiction game. I intend to start writing it up as a sample scenario later on today or tomorrow. I have written to Games Workshop to request addresses of people who publish Role Playing

Games, although I'm not sure whether they'll reply to me.

Walked around Royston for about twenty minutes looking for the Star Wars magazine and a magazine on R.P.G.s. Didn't find either, and as a result I will have to wait until next week to see if I can pick them up then. As a result of this I had no time to go to the bookshop to order a copy of the public enquiry into Strangeways. It's not that serious though, as the nurse said that she could order it for me on her break (they haven't sussed yet - I hope they don't), or failing that I may be able to order it through a friend on another Bungalow.

Once I do get hold of a copy of this enquiry, I am intending to write up my own opinion as 'Ten Years After 002'. This will be printed elsewhere, but I have written another letter to A.K. Distribution, to ask them if they would be willing to help distribute it for me. Posted out all the mail I put into envelopes yesterday. I used the last few copies of the R.P.R. leaflet, which makes it important that I get the next run next week.

Went to the Post Office as well, and bought some envelopes, which is important to the running of this group, as I had recently run out. Without envelopes nothing gets done.

I'm still waiting for a response from Chatto & Windus Press. I suspect that the manuscript must have got there yesterday or today, although I've received no phone call. I gave them my phone number so that they could ring me up requesting return postage when they read it. I've still heard nothing.

The last thing to document today is that I phoned Peace News as regards advertising. They asked me to leave my phone number as they are currently changing their views on advertising, etc. I'm hoping that their rates aren't going to vary too much, as I am poor and things are very tight.

Having said that, there's not really much more to write today. The plan with the hospital poetry pamphlet is still going ahead, and I am still waiting for a reply from the Princes Trust. There may have been a deterioration in my writing style today. This I have to put down to yesterday's injection. It hurt. What's more it messed up my thinking. They give me this injection, because they say I am "not capable of making a decision" about whether or not I want their brainwashing chemicals. They increased my injection after I wrote *How to Make a Petrol Bomb*, and again when I got into the Association of Autonomous Astronauts, so they can't say it isn't political. I am a political prisoner of the Rebeccaist uprising. In twenty years time it will look like a travesty that I have been deliberately set up by the State on the basis of what I think. My views will not have become outdated, they will slowly become culturally acceptable, in this I will be helping the prostitutes. This is where my writing will effect change.

But for the time being I stay locked up, running the Guerilla Press on the basis of what is right; misunderstood, but actively going out to organise a possibility of organised revolution, built from the ashes of the early '90s. For the moment society hasn't grown to accept the views of the Guerilla Press, but in the future that will change. We are the people who will effect change, and we will be there in the future when this revolution becomes reality.

For the moment we struggle. But this struggle will become the movement of the future. We are this country's only active revolutionary guerrilla unit, and we will remain so until such time as the left catch up. For liberation, for revolution, for the future. The retaliation of the people will never end.

5/3/99.

No headaches today. Today has been very quiet, although I have got a lot done. Received the manuscript to an old novel today: a science fiction novel that I called *Picasso Nine*. It has apparently been declined because of the spelling mistakes, although he has offered me web space for Science Fiction. I will send him the manuscript to 'e'.

No mail was collected today, and Dad didn't come, so as a result I have no post to write about, other than the post I prepared today. And I did prepare quite a lot of post today.

Went through the Writers & Artists Yearbook 1998 last night, and discovered quite a few interesting addresses. As a result I have been addressing envelopes. I have posted about ten envelopes, each enclosing one copy of the Demands list, two copies of the 'e' leaflet, two copies of the Guerilla Press leaflet, one copy of the duplicate letter and an S.A.E. I await copies of my change of address leaflet: I printed it out on the computer earlier, and I have sent it to the printers to photocopy along with the original of my headed notepaper to the new address in London. This leaflet I intend to put in every mailout. It explains what Marylin has been doing, without mentioning names, and then explains that the solicitor address is now obsolete, and that people should write to my London address to send mail. I am finding it difficult to afford stamps again.

I am now writing another book. This book is to be a compilation of three essays which are erotic. The first is to be a Science Fiction novel that I was writing, and I will complete it later as an erotic essay. The second essay will be 'Girlschool', which is an erotic essay that I wrote last year, and the last essay will be one about prostitution that I am writing now. Although I have no title to this last essay, I am currently planning to finish it and turn it into a stageplay. That'll be when I get out, although I am planning to have fun writing it tonight.

175

Mum phoned last night, saying that she'd received the card I sent via her to my brother for his birthday. I am happy that she's received it, and I intend to buy him a computer book in Cambridge next week. He spent his birthday watching a play. It sounds like he'd had a nice day, and it sounds like he is happy. That's just about all I have to write today, although I expect some mail tomorrow or later tonight.

7/3/99.

Had another headache last night; took two paracetamols. No headaches yet today, though. Work on the 'elbiB' started today. More tomorrow.

8/3/99.

The article on the following pages appeared in a paper called 'Parasol Post', which I received through the post last night (it was brought here by my Dad). This caused me some confusion, as it was not me who wrote it. It is very cliched Marylin, and I am definite that she wrote it.

As for their saying that my work is "decidedly dodgy," I wrote to them last night sending them a copy of the Demands list. The 'Statement ov Intent' was, admittedly, a bit homophobic, but I have since publicly renounced it with a leaflet.

Anyway, nothing much has happened today, except that work continues on the elbiB. This is a mass project, and I am expecting to finish it next year. It has to be good practise for my writing, and it seems like a project that has to be taken all the way through. I am finding it quite difficult so far, but I think it will be something that will be worthwhile in the long run. Anyway, 1 think it will have some status attributed to it when it is finished.

Phoned Chatto & Windus this morning. They are interested in Book 1, although they are not so interested in the elbiB. I feel very tired at the moment. The elbiB seems to be taking it out of me.

9/3/99 - 11/3/99.

The next two days of this diary are taken up with an article that was printed in the Situationist magazine, Parasol Post. This article was apparently signed by myself, that is, it was signed by my own name, and was followed with a statement that my work was 'dodgy' due to the homophobic nature of the woman who wrote it (here referred to as 'Marylin'). This article did cause me some upset, although that soon passed.

12/3/99.

Little is happening at the present moment, as I am hard at typing the elbiB. Even so, some interesting mail came this morning.

Marylin is still threatening to take me to court. She wrote me a letter (received this morning), which basically rants on about how I am a "hippocrit," which I suppose I am. Nothing really important will come out of this, although I have deleted her from my contacts list.

Another comrade wrote this morning, Mike. I thought his letter was really nice. He basically stated that he supported my hunger strike, and that to him it represented misery. I wrote back to him to tell him that the hunger strike has now ended.

A letter from Games Workshop as well. They are saying that they can't give me the addresses of people who might publish my game, as the only games they sell are those commissioned by themselves. I will get back to them, sending them a copy of 'e'. I'll also send copies to the Science Fiction contacts in the Writers & Artists Yearbook.

It was quite nice to find so many new contacts in the Yearbook. I found a whole section on 'Societies', so I wrote a few letters: one to the 'Society of Indexers' about the R.P.R., and one to some 'International Philosophical Society'. These people are apparently dedicated to the discussion of philosophy that would otherwise never be discussed. I still await news from Chatto & Windus about my book. Still no news from the Animal Liberation Front about the M.M.R. project, so I have written to the Anarchist Communist Federation instead.

The only problem this week has been getting into Royston. I have 200 photocopies waiting at the printers, and I haven't had the chance to pick them up yet. This is causing more aggro. I have the money to pay for them, but I am in debt. I really don't know what to do about it yet. It looks like I may have to wait until next week.

The rest of the news is that I found out the date of my exam for the G.C.S.E. Psychology course. It is June the 8th, so I have some revision to do now. I am sitting the higher paper, and I feel confident that I will pass. I just have to do some reading now; I can do it though.

Planning another mailout to contacts when the photocopying comes back. I might write to Marylin to say sorry. elbiB.

13/3/99.

The elbiB continues. Nowadays I am spending most of my time on the computer, getting into typing the Bible backwards. Today I have been sorting out my graphics.

There's this bloke on another Bungalow, and firstly he's a Jehovah's Witness, and secondly he's into photography. So I have told him that I am typing the first Bible for the internet. He seems impressed. I've told him that if he can take 1500 photographs of Gargoyles in Cambridge, then I would be happy to pay for films and development, and to get them put onto C.D. ROM. He thinks this is a good idea.

The thing is, if I have all these Gargoyles on C.D. ROM, it might be a good idea to copy them, and sell, say, '1500 Gargoyles for the Internet'. It might be a good idea, and it might pay for the elbiB project.

I still haven't got my photocopying back from the printers yet. I gave Janet £10 to go into town and pick it up this morning, but by the time she had got to the printers they were closed.

Granny came to see me today, and gave me £20 and 40 cigarettes. This was instead of Dad visiting, so I have paid off my debts and I intend to put some money into the bank. The only other thing that I feel necessary to document today, is that I am beginning to feel depressed. There seems to be nothing in my life to continue for. I do not feel suicidal, but I do feel that I have lost the most important years of my life. I have done nothing to deserve being locked up in this hospital for the past four years. I feel that I could have overthrown the State if I had been left to my own liberty. Instead the psychiatric control system has screwed me up beyond all recognition. To make matters worse, I still seem to have no support from the left.

Because of this I now feel like wrapping up the campaign and reviving the Guerilla Press at a later date. At the moment, the elbiB is the most important project. Who knows? It might lead somewhere eventually. But as it continues I am practising evil; now in the belief that evil can work for the purposes of the greater good.

14/3/99.

No entry.

15/3/99.

Janet has got her hands on a Pagan magazine called 'Beltane Fire'. It is an interesting magazine, photocopied, and I have seen a couple of things in it which I have gone for. The first is advertising. The cost to put an advert in Beltane Fire is only £2.00, so I have sent them a copy of an advert for the R.P.R. The next thing of interest in that magazine is that it listed a couple of 'Vampyre Societies'. Being in the process of typing the Bible backwards, it seems that this might be what I do next. So I have written to them, sending some money.

Marylin wrote to me the other day, ranting on about how I have "stolen her idea" for the free postage scam, and accusing me of having stolen her painting. Obviously I haven't, but the staff demanded that I let them read her letter.

Things in the hospital at the moment are going slowly. It has now taken me over a week to get into Royston to pick up my photocopying. At this rate the printers are going to start disliking me. I still haven't had the chance to pick up my library book. Even so, I might get a trip into Cambridge on Thursday. I have some money since Granny's visit, and I have cancelled the cheques I sent to A.K. Distribution and Raido A.A.A.; and this will leave me with quite a lot of money to spend. I have nothing in particular that I want to print at the moment, so I can spend. I want to buy a book on Enochian Magick and some Sodom for the purposes of typing the elbiB. I also want to buy a present for my brother. At the same time I need to buy pens and envelopes, etc.

This is Monday's entry, but at present there is little to write. I await my mail, but it might not arrive. I intend to finish today's entry later tonight.

6.45 pm: The elbiB project continues. I intend to send the work so far to pornography; to say "here's the elbiB - I need some photographs to turn this into the Satanic Website." The plan was to use photographs of Gargoyles. Thinking about it, I would prefer to turn it into something pornographic: the elbiB is Satanic, and I feel that pornography would be appropriate in this situation.

This website, regardless of what graphics I eventually use, will be linked in with Demands of the Cross. But I am really looking for photographs of a pretty seventeen year old with dreadlocks, lace mini-dress, woollen socks and Combat Boots. Having said this, and having included this in the second Volume of C.C.A., I feel that I should escalate this idea to the fullest of my ability, or once more be accused of hypocrisy. We have eventually been converted into Satanism; and the views hereof are nothing more than the escalation of the evil of the Bardier Rebeccaism.

16/3/99.

After a week of waiting, I eventually got into Royston today to pick up my photocopying. Therefore I have not had time to write to pornography. I might get on to it later; otherwise tomorrow.

I have asked the printers for a quote on 100 pamphlets and 600 double-sided leaflets. This pamphlet will be the manuscript to *Propaganda Groups*, and will be the first publication under the R.P.R. I intend to print these as a trade edition, and to keep 20 copies after sending the rest to radical bookshops and library agencies. This publication will carry the number 0001 on the inside front cover, and an explanation of this as the first publication under the Radical Presses Register. This will essentially explain the idea, as well as giving an address for further information.

At the same lime I intend to print 600 copies of another leaflet, this explaining the R.P.R., and trying to sell the book. This will be sent out with copies of the pamphlet, and also to people who are involved with publishing, indexing etc. So, that's the plan so far. I'll keep people informed.

No mail arrived today. I am currently unaware as to whether my solicitor has been allowing me to use her address since Marylin threw her tantrum. Either way I am not getting much mail from either address, so I am waiting for some mail to come via my contact address in London. Still, things are moving far too slowly to be comfortable. And I don't really expect things to pick up very soon.

Out of passing it is worth a mention that I saw the dentist today. A chip fell out of my front tooth, so I made an appointment to see the hospital dentist. It didn't go as well as I thought it would.

Firstly he scraped away at my front tooth, until it was almost gone, then he drilled. Then he started scraping again. Then he drilled again. All this lasted about an hour, when I had only come to see him with a tiny chip in my front tooth.

Anyway, they kept sucking, drilling, sucking, water squirting things into my mouth and drilling. After a while he took out a piece of what looked like cotton, and stuck it into my teeth. Then he started to break it: whilst it was still in my mouth! If this wasn't frightening enough, they then started putting an orange thing in front of my face, and a strange blue light into my mouth, that made my head vibrate. Ruling class snobby tossers! Never again!

17/3/99.

An uneventful day today in terms of things happening in the hospital. No mail and no trips out, but two ducks have made a new home in the pond and we also have frogs. Although I have received no mail for the past few days, I spent this morning working flat out an a mailout, and had a nap in the afternoon.

The first of the letters I sent today was quite a large thing, a printout of the current work on the elbiB, which I sent to pornography. I sent it to the computer pornography magazine (a huge coincidence in the way the address corresponded), asking if they could sort me out with 1500 gif. files of one model (wearing a short lace skirt and a leather jacket). I enclosed an S.A.E. and I await a reply.

The next letter was also quite big. It was a copy of the Science Fiction game that I wrote a while ago; I found a single photocopy stashed away somewhere. So I sent it to that person who was interested in putting 'Picasso Nine' on the internet, asking him if he was interested in the game if I programmed it up in JavaScript. Again I enclosed an S.A.E. and await a reply.

On top of this I spent this morning writing a duplicate letter to everyone on the contacts list concerning the R.P.R. I have decided to print the manuscript to *Propaganda Groups* as a pamphlet, and I sent out a letter about that, and a leaflet about the recent change of address. I can just about afford to print *Propaganda Groups*, and I feel that this would be a good idea to set up the R.P.R. If there is one first title with an R.P.R. number, then I can send it to librarians and indexers with a copy of a leaflet and a duplicate letter. Still, this is going to take some time and a lot of thought, so I'll write more as it comes together.

No work on the elbiB today.

Incidentally, I noticed yesterday, as I was in Royston, that the bookshop that grassed me up over the 'V.M.P. Statement ov Intent' (see Volume 1) has closed down. In doing this, the bloke who stirred it up over my publications has run off with quite a lot of money that I put down as a deposit on a book. So! This could finally be my opportunity to take the bastard to court and get my own back. I intend to write to my solicitor tomorrow.

18/3/99.

The sad news today is that I have started to go deaf. I got out of bed this morning, and there was a constant humming sound in my left ear. It hasn't gone away all day, and it has seriously affected my concentration. It has also affected my hearing.

After years of hearing nothing but verbal abuse, at last, this might end. I actually feel very upset that I will lose all my friends, and I have started to cry. After so many years of this abuse; why should it be like this? That said, I can only find some advantages in this. There will be no accusations. There will be no one telling me that I shouldn't write. Above all there will be no authority.

Asides from that, things have been fairly productive today. That is aside from the constant humming in my ear affecting my concentration. I received the photocopying through the post this morning, which was nice. I also received something from Hare Krishna, about an event that I won't be able to attend until I am deaf.

Started putting together *Propaganda Groups* as a pamphlet. This is going OK, apart from the constant humming and the fact that I don't have as much money in the bank as I thought I did. Even so, finances are about sorted, with the next week's allowance free to spend on postage.

Spending a lot of time revising for my psychology exam at the moment. I would ideally like to continue with psychology to do a degree in the subject. Still, I feel that I cannot write much more tonight, as the humming in my left ear is very annoying indeed.

On reflection, it may not be the best move to do a degree course. Without it I have all the time in the world, and I wish to work on the R.P.R. and the elbiB.

19/3/99.

Yesterday's entry might have been premature, as the humming in my ear has gone today, and I feel a lot better. Did no psychology revision today, as I went to a concert and finished typing out *Propaganda Groups*.

The concert was in Cambridge, and was organised by education (hospital O.T.s). Although the entire gig was very good, the first bit was very good indeed. It was called 'Dark Matter', by a bloke named Dave Davey. It was a session about space with a professor talking about the cosmos, whilst this bloke just sat there with a keyboard making strange space noises.

After the gig I took his phone number, and I intend to phone him on Monday. I would like to set up some sort of management for him, offering him some time in a recording studio to do a benefit for the Guerilla Press. Whatever happens, this is going to take a lot more time.

Received a copy of a magazine from the Highgate Vampyre Society today. Although I haven't yet read it, I look at it with interest, as it was in Highgate that I sent back the crucifixion of Jesus Christ. I may wish to write something on the subject; there are a lot of dodgy things that happen in the Whittington Hospital, and getting involved with this lot may seem like a good *move*.

Marylin sent another letter through my solicitor, but my solicitor is saying that it's best if I don't read her letters any more. She seems to think there is a possibility that Marylin might sue, but that this isn't apparent yet. For the time being she says that she will still forward my mail.

As I sit here and write this, the head staff of Rehab turns up. He's saying that he will come to the next Community Meeting, and he has asked me to compile a list of questions from the patients, so that he can "have something to say." Through constantly protesting my sanity, I have earned respect. I now seem to have become the patients' representative. I have been solely at the head of the protest about Rehab money. I feel that the secret is to earn respect, if you are ever to become a successful revolutionary.

20/3/99.

Spent today doing very little, waiting for my Dad to come down. When I did get down to getting something done, I sent copies of the Science Fiction game to a number of addresses that I found in the Writers & Artists Yearbook 1998. Some post today, but it was mainly from people who had sent copies of their stuff via a different address, and some magazines.

Nothing from the A.C.F. to the London address; it now looks like the M.M.R. project has to be kept on hold for a while, at least until I am in London. I'm now considering not printing the leaflet, not just now at least, but instead printing the pamphlet and buying another ink cartridge. I may have to do this to afford more stamps. Things are very tight financially just at the moment.

21/3/99.

Sunday is usually the day for doing things that you would not want to do in the week. Today I am making my bed, washing my clothes, cooking a meal and having a shave. Although things are running very slowly, it still looks like things with the C.C.A. are starting to get going. It's just little things, like signals, making me think that people are beginning to listen to what I have to say.

There is usually a church service on Sunday, although I don't feel that I'll be going today. But I'll be typing the elbiB later. The procedure for getting to church in the hospital always causes a headache. We have to find a member of staff to take us over there; there usually isn't a member of staff available; then I usually have to walk over there with a 'personality disorder' ward; then I have to walk all the way down to the locked ward and navigate my way through a maze of corridors, eventually to find the 'chapel room'. There are always a number of people there, worshipping the lord in differing states of delusion; and the service is usually very boring.

In this hell hole, people still seem to believe that Christ will save them. Christ wouldn't be able to find his way into Holland House, even if he did come back to walk on the Earth.

The thing is, I can't seem to get it out of my head that I may be the second coming of the messiah. The crucifixion: Jesus must have done something equally as controversial in his lifetime to have gone down as such an important martyr on the Cross. I believe that what I did was the same thing, but in a current-day setting. But surely the crucifixion of Christ was wrong? Not if it worked for the greater good; and it was the crucifixion that resulted in the I.R.A. cease-fire in Northern Ireland.

Unfortunately the press don't seem to be able to see this, going on and on with their perpetual slander. Even so, I see it as this controversy that implicates me as the second messiah. I have had disciples. Does this seem arrogant? Maybe so but, if I am wrong, which I accept I may be, then surely that must be a symptom of the so-called mental illness that I supposedly suffer from.

4.30 pm: Work on the elbiB is going very slowly indeed. In one sense, I don't want to continue work on it. But another part of me says I have all the time in the world, and that it is right to continue with it. So the decision is to do at least an hour each morning.

I did eventually get to church this morning. Mary was doing the service, and it was quite enjoyable. Even so, I have decided to worship Satan in Corpus Christi. It just seems like the best thing to do. As well as which, it's a lot more fun.

Now to change the subject. I sent six copies of the Science Fiction game to different organisations last night; each letter containing a stamped addressed envelope and a number of leaflets. Sent two to science fiction societies (found them in the Writers & Artists Yearbook), one to a publisher, one to a Games publisher, and one to a science fiction magazine. I will probably get a lot of them back, but I am still hoping that a few people will be interested in the game. If so I will send them a copy each. But I don't really think that many people will be, judging by the response I have had so far.

I still have to reply to the Highgate Vampyre Society. I wonder if they are interested that it was in the psychiatric hospital in Highgate, that the assassination of Christ took place? He, also, was very controversial.

22/3/99.

With every day that passes, I feel more like doing a runner. I have been locked up since I was seventeen, and I still live on a pittance handed out by my family, and the bank will refuse to give me a loan to set up a business or do anything. I feel as though I am being treated like a child.

What stops me from doing an escape job is this diary and the C.C.A. group. It has stopped me from doing a runner so many times in the past, but I now begin to wonder what more I'd be able to achieve if I wasn't here. The fact is that I am wrongly imprisoned and that I am not insane. The only thing that stops me from absconding is my coming exam. So I have to wait until at least September: they were talking about discharging me at that point anyway. So I play the system with the Guerilla Press.

And on that subject, I took *Propaganda Groups* to the printers today. I can afford to print 100 copies and 200 leaflets, and I have decided to do that, although that means I have to rely on a double dole cheque on Thursday. In the future I want to print 1,000 leaflets solely on the politics of prostitution and the gun, and just send out piles of 20 to different campaigns. Even so, I doubt that I will build much more support than that I already have.

Anyway, that's just about all I have time to write tonight, as not much has actually taken place. More tomorrow.

23/3/99.

Received a letter from Action Against Injustice today, enclosing a questionnaire concerning detention in custody, police bias, etc. Although a lot of it wasn't relevant to my situation, I filled it out making it so. For example, for the question regarding "were your civil rights in custody in any way violated," I responded that the only civil rights awarded to asylum patients is the right to one biased tribunal each year. I sent this back to them with a number of leaflets.

The A.A.I. are actually very controversial amongst the anarchist movement. This started last year with the nationally organised hunger strike. The hunger strike itself was a big success on one level, although I was myself transferred back to a locked ward because of it. Anyway, it was after the hunger strike that a number of anarchist groups claimed that, in actual fact, it wasn't the A.A.I. who did most of the organisational work at all. They claimed that it was actually them. Anyway, shortly after the event, a number of groups sent literature to anarchist groups, saying that the A.A.I. were ex-Militant, bureaucratic and totally obsessed with their own movement. This literature went on that the A.A.I. were calling meetings at short notice when it suited them, and so on. No one is really sure where it goes from here, but the A.A.I. have since been boycotted on a large scale by the anarchists. However, it has always been the stance of the C.C.A. that, whoever is helping us out, we will support, regardless of what the anarchist scene is saying.

On to other news, I have still heard no news from this keyboard player that I saw in Cambridge. I was thinking of organising a benefit gig, or possibly offering some sort of small-scale management project but, having no money, this is going to be difficult. I am thinking of asking him for one of his C.D.s and, if I can make an independent claim for D.L.A. benefit, then I may be able to get something together for Cross Bootlegs Distribution. This will be another project, but at the moment I can only afford to run the Guerilla Press.

Janet cooked me a meal this evening. Unfortunately she let the potatoes boil dry until there was an actual fire, and she overcooked the sweetcorn. My girlfriend must come close to being the planet's worst cook. An Interstellar Cabinet Gorgon could cook better food. Fortunately Janet hasn't been able to contact them yet, but if she keeps writing letters to pen-pal groups, then it won't take long.

24/3/99.

No post came today. Again the staff forgot to collect it. Received a phone call from Dave Davey, the keyboard player today. I'm discussing some sort of record deal type scene. The plan is, once I have found the music I like from him (he does different stuff), I am going to print a short run of C.D.s and a black and white pamphlet to go with it, and distribute a leaflet to the Free Information Network about his stuff. There is a possibility that I might be able to use my Dad's recording studio to get stuff done. Eventually, if I can earn money from it, I may be able to distribute a proper C.D. with a full colour glossy booklet, but let's see what happens. The Cestre Cantre Advocation are becoming the Cross Bootlegs Group, and I am becoming a manager.

The rest of the day has been spent in revision, and I have started to address envelopes for next week's mailout. Hopefully there will be some more post tomorrow, and I will be able to write a longer entry.

25/3/99.

My mental illness lasted five years. I am sane now, and have been since first coming into mental hospital. Being held in mental hospital, against my will, has made me a political prisoner. It has also made me very bitter. It isn't just that they have no right to keep me on a locked ward; it is also that they have no right to keep me in hospital at all when I am sane. Even so, I acknowledge that at one time I was mentally ill. My mental illness was started by a prostitution racket on the Convoy. This is how it happened.

Jenny, an ex-girlfriend, started on the road under the impression that the most popular job on the Convoy was prostitution. She met Colin, who had already decided that he wanted to be a pimp. Therefore he offered to lend Jenny some money if she slept with him. As soon as she accepted, Colin used his influence in the Oxford squat scene to make her very popular as a prostitute.

A week later, Colin had got the money together, and had arranged a date with Jenny. After going to a gig, and getting her just a bit drunk, he went back to his van, as you do, to fuck her and to discuss lending her £2,000, which she had already agreed to pay back through prostitution. Whilst there, alone, Colin spiked the first bit of a spliff with Spanish Fly. Getting into a frenzy of sex, she agreed to his deal of accepting £40 for each fuck, and to pay Colin £30 of it each time, to pay him back. Then they fucked. So Jenny had, at the age of sixteen, started as Colin's first whore.

Being popular under the influence of Colin's standing on the circuit in Oxford, Jenny didn't find it hard to find enough men to screw. At this point she was having a lot of fun: sleeping around, snorting cocaine, and becoming popular for it. What she didn't know was that her popularity had been set up, by Colin, in order for the Convoy to set up prostitution.

Things escalated quite quickly and, before she had paid back the

186

£2,000, her van was already being used as a brothel by Convoy prostitutes being used by a group of Hells Angels called Oxford Road Rats. At this point she was already developing a taste for cocaine. The Road Rats had developed a liking for her.

As Jenny became more popular, the Convoy in Oxford decided that prostitution would be a good way of making some money to get into cocaine. The situation escalated, Jenny's debt to Colin slowly getting bigger as her addiction grew. And the Road Rats saw a good scene going down.

It was OK before the Road Rats got on but, as they got into the scene, more and more threats started circulating. Threats of influential members of the squat scene being shot dead, threats of dodgy cocaine getting around, and lots of Spanish Fly. No one seemed to be able to get around it, as the Road Rats carried guns and had contacts with Hells Angels. Anyone who tried to do anything about it was shot. Jenny got more and more depressed until she was eventually a gibbering wreck, seen by Road Rats to be good for nothing more than screwing thirty men a night in order to feed her cocaine habit.

That's what took place. That's what drove me insane.

26/3/99.

Some interesting mail today. A letter from Advocacy and a letter from hospital complaints. The letter from Advocacy just said that they were still off sick, and the letter from complaints said, again, that there was nothing they could do to help me. Complaints went on to say that, if I wasn't happy with the situation as regards rehab money, which I'm not, then I can contact my funding authority; which I intend to do.

The other letter I received today was from the London Vampyre Group. They sent me a number of leaflets and some membership details. Interestingly enough, they are also trying to distribute some information on what they are doing. This gives me an idea.

What I intend to do, is to print a duplicate letter for Wednesday's mailout. In this letter, I am going to ask everyone, in particular the groups, of which there are a few, if they would be interested in being on a printed contacts list. I will also ask if anyone wishes to be taken off the mailing list. At the same time as writing this, I intend to offer mailouts of newsletters etc., stuff that costs 50p or something, in return for a donation of £5.00. That way I can afford to get copies of newsletters, etc., from people such as the numerous Vampyre Groups, and distribute them to the contacts list. I hope that this will be productive.

I cooked a meal for Janet tonight. Stir fry with peppers and bean sprouts. Apart from that nothing has happened today. The next entry is Saturday.

28/3/99.

Bad news with the technology side of the Guerilla Press. The computer's gone and blown up. No more duplicate letters. No more pamphlets. Nothing. I turned the machine on, and it wouldn't load. I'm not exactly sure what's gone wrong with it, but it causes a massive problem. And I'm not sure exactly what to do about it, although I intend to go to the computer shop where I bought it and ask them.

The worst thing about it is that I haven't yet been able to tell my Dad, who bought the computer for me in the first place. I will have to try and tell him during the week. Even so, I have to look at it as if it has its positive aspects. But for the time being I'm stuck.

So the next thing I have to do is to make a new claim for Disability Living Allowance. It hasn't been given to the patients for a couple of years now: the dole decided that the patients of this hospital wouldn't be entitled to it, so they stopped D.L.A. payments to the entire hospital. The thing is that I am going to need D.L.A. if I am going to be able to sort the computer problem, and also if I am going to manage the keyboard musician who I have been speaking to on the phone this week.

What I intend to do, therefore, is to make a claim for D.L.A. from my Dad's address in London. When that comes through, I can take the dole book to the Post Office in Royston and cash it there. They will ask me for a change of address statement, so I will give them an abbreviated version of the hospital address. After that, all I have to remember, is to keep the whole thing a secret.

Some interesting mail yesterday, most of which I still have to reply to. Letter from the British library, saying that they are interested in the R.P.R. scheme, but that they don't think that I have kept them fully informed of the moves of the Guerilla Press. I actually think I have done, but there may be some confusion with the titles that I put on the back of the *Discharge Not Depixol* leaflet. I listed *Prostitution*, which hasn't yet gone to print, as being one of our titles. This was formerly entitled *How to Make a Petrol Bomb* and printed on a photocopier, but I sent them few copies. The next title was *Propaganda Groups* and, as documented, this pamphlet comes out next week. So I'll have to write to them telling them this. I am assuming that what they are saying is that they want to be kept more informed on the movements of the R.P.R.; but without a computer, it is very difficult to do this.

The next letter was from a comrade called Sam, who runs a small scale record distribution scene. He sent me a pile of leaflets, which I have put in next week's mailout, which I like. He also sent me a letter, essentially saying that he was on my side over this scene with Marylin, which was nice, and enquiring about whether *Evil Things* was going to print. Unfortunately it isn't but, again, I will send him a copy of *Propaganda Groups* instead.

There was also a letter from Animal, which was nice, because I had actually been under the impression that they had been ignoring my mail. It was only a short letter, however, saying that they didn't agree with the politics of Advocism, which wasn't really a surprise. I'll write back to them later on: it is going to be a letter-writing day.

The next letter was a prospectus from the University of North London. I haven't had time to study it properly yet, but it looks like the course to take is the same one that I was doing when I attempted suicide. That's the City & Guilds course in Sound and Recording. As a last note to Sunday morning's entry: today I must wash my clothes, and do some more revision.

8.10 pm: With the computer down, I have to start on the next project. I have decided to use the opportunity to work on the book about the Vectron Mars Project, and to revise psychology (I've done no revision today). But the next project I intend to get into is drawing the roughs for the pornographic Tarot.

This Tarot will be Satanic, not just in that the drawings will be taken from my favourite magazine (mentioned in Book 2), but also in that I will be working on an accompanying book, to describe the tarot in Satanism. It was the Tarot that got me into Satanism in the first place.

Initially the drawings will be roughs: drawn in pencil and gone over in pen. I intend to buy pencils if I can get into Royston tomorrow. The first card I will draw will be 'the lovers', but I will really need to buy myself a copy of the Book of Thoth when I can afford it. But this first card will be a lesbian scene. I intend to get the roughs turned into colour photographs or paintings by a publisher. So - until the computer's fixed: the Tarot. Hence this diary will be a chronology of the Satanic Tarot and dreams.

29/3/99.

Got the printing back from Royston today. One hundred pamphlets, and two hundred leaflets. Most of the leaflets are gone already, sent out with the mailout I posted earlier. Called in at the library and picked up a book on the Tarot, which looks interesting, if I ever get to read it. Also called into the computer shop. The good news is that they say they can fix the problem. The bad news is that they are charging £25.00 per hour to do it.

Anyway, I have another headache coming, and I just want to go to bed again. I will write a longer entry tomorrow.

30/3/99.

Sent another twelve copies of *Propaganda Groups* this morning, as well as sending some to the legal deposit places. I have now sent out about half of them, but I am slightly uncertain about where I should send the rest. But I now feel that something is going to happen, whether that be something to do with the Guerilla Press setting up as an enterprise (situationist counter-capitalist), or the R.P.R. Whatever happens, I have used my address in London for all of it. So I have to wait now. The next project is to get D.L.A., and to set up managing Dave Davey, and to set up for the pamphlet released on the Summer Solstice (Cease-fire).

Saw my solicitor today, and the meeting was a bit weird. On the one hand she discussed my Tribunal, which seems to be "looking rosy" in her words. On the other hand, she will not acknowledge the situation as regards the broadcasting of what I am thinking, mainly by the B.B.C. This essentially means that one door has closed, and any legal case I might theoretically have had against the media treating me absolutely like a total pile of shit, isn't upheld as a case in law. Therefore I am given no choice about continuing to run the C.C.A. - despite the blatant disapproval of my parents and the trouble I am getting into with the staff. It makes me wonder what the State actually mean by the term "justice."

As I still have some space to write in tonight's entry, I feel that it could be appropriate to discuss my involvement with the assassination of Christ. My moves would have been entirely different if I hadn't been given that assignment; and I have come to believe that I have been set up by the F.B.I. It may be the case that the Church of Satan are a front for the F.B.I., and that in upholding that assignment, I am a part of that scene, but I have since come to the belief that the crucifixion was wrong.

The situation at the time was that I was an active paramilitary. I had been working extensively to train the prostitutes in guerrilla warfare, and had been the idea and the Godfather behind the Strangeways riots. At the time I met P'tou, I had been in London, making the speech that started the London Poll Tax riots, without a face mask. Things went really well, and after spending a couple of days with my Dad in London, I met this woman whilst getting on the bus back to Swansea.

As she had given me her address, I went up to see her a couple of weeks later. Whilst the story of what took place could easily take another book, she basically gave me an extreme assignment involving joining Satanism. If I hadn't have met her, I would have done something entirely different since then. Anyway, the assignment involved joining Satanism, going into hospital, and getting into a "bizarre ritual," involving making a druid cross on supernatural oaths. This basically sent it back into the past,

190

through the assassins cordor, back to Judas. This was a deliberate plot to kill Christ.

Whatever the excuses, I have since learned that this was the international signal for I.R.A. cease-fire, as I have mentioned before. All the same, I have felt guilty ever since. If I hadn't done that, I would have led the bikers into revolution. I really believe that. But since joining Satanism, everything has gone wrong. After the influence I had due to Strangeways, I now struggle to run the Guerilla Press. This may be because it wasn't directly a threat, or because of the abuse from the press, but I believe that it was due to the crucifixion, and the fact that it was my fault, ten years ago. All I can believe now, is that the struggle continues. I try to repent to Christ, but there is so much against me, and my alter-egos don't help. The future now is in the Guerilla Press, and where to take it when I eventually find myself being discharged.

31/3/99.

There no longer seems to be a reason to assassinate Bill Clinton. The way I have been flirting with Janet; well, I think I should discuss something else Since I split up with Beelzebub, there have been no riots in this country.

Went to the library today, to ask if they kept newspaper records. As it happens, in Royston they don't. Anyway, I have put in a request for articles from tabloid papers on the subject of the Angry Brigade 1972-1984. They say they are going to write to me when they come in. This is so that I can compile a pamphlet of newspaper clippings on the Angry Brigade, to release on the Summer Solstice of this year. Next year is the big one. I will be absconding to be at Stonehenge in the year 2000.

Anyway, there was no mail today and, apart from writing letters to the Stonehenge Campaign, Sabotage Editions and Radical Bookseller, nothing else of significance has happened with the Guerilla Press today.

1/4/99.

Book 1 has been rejected by Chatto & Windus. "Just too controversial." I feel utterly depressed by the verdict; everything in my life since Strangeways has gone wrong. I blame it on Satanism. It was whilst Strangeways was going on that I was forced into Devil Worship.

Tonight I burn the Bible. It was the Bible that crashed my computer, Jesus Christ who fucked my life. I feel close to tears, and this sacrilege is the only option as far as I am concerned. I wish to escalate my worship of Beelzebub.

Furthermore it occurs to me that I wouldn't be here if I hadn't broken my spine. Is what I did so unjustified given the circumstances? In my life I have only tried to do my best for the people I respect: the downtrodden and the exploited. I have done my utmost to fight for the liberation of the prostitutes and all those incarcerated under the laws of the Bible. All this exploitation perpetuated in the name of Christ. Tonight I burn the Bible.

Today I received a letter from the National Extension College. They want my 'Student Candidate Number' and my 'Examination Centre Number', or else my coursework could be "in jeopardy." I have been on to the hospital teachers all day; apparently they need to get in contact with the local college before they will be able to find the relevant information for me. I just hope they can get it together in time. I have to admit that I am fairly worried about the exam.

Went to the exhibition in the main hospital building today. It was an interesting exhibition: a collection of the art and photography of patients involved in the project group over the last few months. I was in charge of signing people in, taking the names of staff and patients that attended. A good friend was given his City & Guilds certificate, and all in all it was quite a nice day. All the same, I am still feeling depressed.

The system of justice in this country is seriously flawed. If a sane person, such as myself, can be incarcerated and forced with mind altering medication, under these pretences, then something is seriously wrong. Above that, if psychology can be so ignorant of the facts of the situation as exists in my case, then something seriously has to change. If this country's alternative scene can sit and watch such a miscarriage of justice on this scale, it makes you wonder as to the nature of the human mind. It poses the question: is human nature really good? If the Bible can dictate the very nature of human survival, then how can the nature of what we are told to believe is good, be respected?

I would really like to see a situation whereby the Bible is overthrown; where prostitution is accepted to the extent that it is not only legal, but also popular. This is the purpose behind the Cross of Valhalla, the purpose behind my work, and the reason I worship Beelzebub. Society will learn, I hope. But to those ends, tonight I burn the Bible.

2/4/99.

Burning the Bible last night was difficult. But I burned it, and it made a great connotation with the ritual I have been working until now. Last night was the final ritual. This is to uphold the relevance of the Irish situation, if such a thing exists.

It is on that note that I make retort to the critique raised by the opponents of the war I fight. If certain individuals and the press, who collectively term themselves "counter-revolutionaries" (which they are), ask "what have the Guerilla Press ever done to support guerrillas?," the response is simple. What I am doing, single handedly, is the escalation of my own actions of bombing Downing Street, and Strangeways. I believe that it was my own actions in these attacks that directly led to the 'Good Friday Agreements'. The role I play now is to keep the movements of the anti-Poll Tax resistance and Strangeways alive and in context with the 'Peace Talks'. I believe that I represent a third way; an alternative to the nations disputes of Nationalism and Loyalism as they exist across the water. The third way is not to dictate peace; rather to let the revolution take its natural course. The revolution is obvious. But I don't write it here.

As the ritual has became an established part of my cell, the war in Yugoslavia rages. I take this as an opportunity to take advantage of the media perpetuation of the monitoring of thought. I make myself controversial by reading Volume 2 of Karl Marx (*Das Kapital*).

Obtained the phone number of the dole office in charge of disability. I intend to claim from my Dad's address in London, and change my registered address at the Post Office in Royston when I go in on Wednesday. It isn't really fraud, as I am entitled to D.L.A. as I am actually disabled. The dole was stopped in the hospital a couple of years ago. I feel fit to take my revenge!

3/4/99.

Nothing happened today, so I feel fit to leave space for a longer entry on Sunday, when I should receive my mail.

4/4/99.

A quiet day today, until my Dad came, bringing me some interesting mail and taking me down the pub. Drank a pint of lager and went back to the hospital, where there was a patients' disco.

The disco was a lot more fun than I thought it was going to be, although the place was crawling with staff. There was some good music, and it was loud, and there were some good people there. Still, it is sad that this is the only opportunity the patients have to interact and enjoy ourselves. I got a bad vibe from a patient who once beat me up, however.

Getting there was more of a problem. Apparently there had to be one staff member to every three patients, and I think that this was the reason for the massive number of nurses to patients. So a number of patients went from Wortham ward, whilst myself and another patient went from this one. We went down to Wortham, and ended up having to wait there for about half an hour before two staff came back from their "break," so that there could be someone on that ward whilst nurses took us to the disco on Clopton ward. Every door we went through had to be locked behind us. This liberty. Because I dare to think.

I have been thinking, most recently, about wrapping up the Guerilla Press. In its place I will be establishing the Betelgeuse Publications Group (under the current Cross Distribution Group), in order to publish Science Fiction and Space Rock (Dave Davey, if he ever gets in touch). This is basically because I currently decide to uphold the I.R.A. Good Friday Agreement in Satanic etiquette, and, as such, have announced a Guerilla Press cease-fire for June 21st. The point is that advocating guerrilla warfare is getting me into trouble; not just in hospital, but also with the press. I believe I have now proven my point, and that it is time to step down. It would be good if I could do this in time with the I.R.A. decommissioning of arms.

Some interest in 'e', and this is one reason why I contemplate Betelgeuse Publications. A letter came through my Dad this afternoon, from some bloke who is interested in the Play Testing side of the idea. Still not sure whether he'd be interested in paying the £20.00 fee I demand for stamps, but if so then this will be the start of the first scenario. I have ideas, but hopefully this bloke will be interested and will spread the idea, making Betelgeuse a workable idea. I'll send him a copy of the rules as soon as I get stamps, and I intend to print the rules for release on 7/8/99. I have to remember to print a preview run; maybe the feedback I get from *Propaganda Groups* will help. I have to take this as being the most important break of the week.

Response from Raido A.A.A. He is saying that he is very busy, and therefore has not had time to reply to me earlier. That seems fair enough, and he sent me a pile of leaflets, which was nice, although I'm sure that the staff are never going to allow me to attend the said conference. Still, if I do get out then I'll be there. There is also a chance that I might get some home leave over that weekend, so I'll make an effort to get there.

Stonehenge campaign newsletter arrived, but still they haven't listed my contact address. This causes me some annoyance. Even so, it is nice that they've sent it to me. Some feedback from a woman who seems fairly together, sending a mailout on the subject of certain situations being misunderstood by the system of psychiatric control. I reply to this mail tomorrow. Tonight I'll watch the T.V.

5/4/99.

Written a short work on the Worship of Beelzebub. As a result I feel too tired to write an entry tonight. I'll write more tomorrow.

6/4/99.

I found an address in yesterday's newspaper, one of the sex shop companies. I have written them a letter asking for some Spanish Fly. If it was Spanish Fly that seduced Jenny into prostitution, and I want to set up my own ring, then I could do worse than to spike Janet. And I am feeling inclined to do that. Here's the plan.

Janet sometimes cooks me a meal; she cooked for me tonight. In return I cook for her. So what I intend to do is invite her over here more often, and start getting her to stay for longer each time, staying for coffee and stuff like that. I might start holding her hand. Anyway, I have today made a claim for D.L.A. So what I am going to do is invite her over for a meal, and spike her with just a little bit of the drug. After that I'm going to offer her money to do some pornographic photographs for me. Then, if she agrees, I'm going to fuck her a lot more. If not then I won't fuck her. She'll agree, I think.

When she's agreed to the photos, I do them in my bedroom, her with one of her cuddly teddy bears, and then get them put on to C.D. ROM by the chemist. Then all I have to do is program the pornographic website. It could make me money. It is a highly dodgy plan, but it gets my sexual fetishes.

The computer is still down. I didn't get to take it into Royston today, but I took it apart, and I think I can get in to take it to the computer shop tomorrow. In the meantime, I am writing a short work on the Worship of Beelzebub. I wrote the first draft yesterday, and I think it is quite good. It is basically a booklet on the magickal seals I use to worship her, and it is that which knackered me out last night. I don't know why, but writing this manuscript has made me feel really tired. Strange!

Anyway, with the computer down, I have decided to write the thing in very neat block capitals. I will send it for publication in that format. Still no word from Dave Davey. I'll write a longer entry tomorrow.

7/4/99.

Depixol is giving me headaches. My doctor asked me to keep a diary of my headaches; and it is after receiving an injection that my headaches return. It is another example of the injustice of my being sectioned that I am forced to take an injection every week. There is nothing wrong with my mental state, and the more I tell them that, the more trouble I find myself in. I have concluded that the most trouble that you can find yourself in, is from telling them that you are sane. It comes down to "lacking insight." And the more I moan, protest to the staff and motivate the anarchists, the less support I have.

If, by any chance, I still have an audience after this much bias from the B.B.C., then they must surely be an audience convinced I am mad. In the long run, I must be persecuted for telling the truth. Those who lack insight are the doctors; they lack insight into what is going on in this country. But it is serious as to where this could lead. If they are monitoring thought upon myself because of Strangeways, who do they blame next time there is a revolt in this country? If the anarchists don't support, then who is there to stop this state from escalating?

My own theory is that the left are actually frightened of supporting the issue. After all, who wants to be set up under State telepathy? An attitude from one of my correspondents was that if the State could monitor thought upon myself, then there would be an immediate end to social crime. This was an attitude from an anarchist; someone who thought he was libertarian.

But the situation continues. If the State are currently monitoring thought upon myself, then it must be for a reason. It would seem obvious that it would be as a form of control, proving it is the problem that is keeping me in psychiatric hospital. And with this lack of support from the left, the situation is more serious. I can only blame the B.B.C. and the F.B.I. for a conspiracy that is because of Strangeways. Anyway, the only thing that I can really consider doing is to continue to run the Guerilla Press; using the situation of the public monitoring of thought in order to demonstrate the procedure of running a propaganda group as a means of resistance, when and if the situation should escalate, this being the purpose of the C.C.A. in printing *Propaganda Groups*. In writing this, it makes me think more in terms of continuing the strategy of my first pamphlet.

Now on to other stuff: I have done no revision at all over the past few days. I need to take it much more seriously, if I am to be in with a chance of passing the exam. At the same time I have to get on to education in order to get my 'Student Identifier' number. I have to do this fast, or otherwise my coursework could be in jeopardy. That and revision, I have to get on to it.

Took the computer in to be sorted this afternoon. Debbie took me in with a hospital car. Nice Drive. Difficult carrying it down the street to get it to the shop, but when I eventually got there, the bloke was quite nice. He said he'd have it fixed by tomorrow. Despite this, I won't be able to pick it up until Saturday; I have got to get transport in and I have to wait to get some money to pay for it.

In the meantime I have been working on my manuscript on Beelzebub. I'm writing it out by hand, carefully. I have now drawn out all the seals I intend to use, and I still have to do a write-up for the seals as they stand, but it's going quite well, although slowly, and slightly tediously. Even so, it is giving me something to do. As well as that, when it's finished, it's likely that I will have something different to get published.

Decided to compile the essays that I've published under the Guerilla Press into one Book, and to try to get it published as *Chaoticism: Book 1, Volume 1, A Manual in Subversion.* It still stands that if I can't get it published, with a disclaimer against arson, then I intend to sell my story to the press to raise the funds to print it. After that I look forward to Broadmoor, although I will forever protest my case that I am sane.

8/4/99.

An interesting day. There was a trip out to Wysing Arts today. For those who don't know, Wysing Arts is a small farm that has been converted into an art studio. It's quite nice down there, and going there is really the main thing that has happened today. All the same, it has been an interesting day.

One of the exhibits was a life-sized church that is made entirely of wood. Jazz took some photos of it, and then we wandered around a bit more, exploring the site. It was a lot of fun.

The booklet on Beelzebub is going to take some more time. I don't really know why I started it, if I can get the computer back on Saturday, Even so, I am told that a new grimoir really has to be written out by hand. Therefore I shall do that, working on it until it is finished. So far it is going quite well. I have now drawn out the seals, and started on the first two pages of text.

I've decided that I don't want to see my psychologist again. I have an appointment for tomorrow, but I don't want to go. He pries into all my secrets, and I don't want him to know about things like Strangeways and the subversion of prostitution at the start of the decade that I was responsible for. It is likely to cause a major problem if I don't attend, but I don't need it anymore. And I have my secrets to protect. Security is more important than anything else, and I can't risk him getting on to Strangeways and the Good Friday agreements.

So the plan is just not to turn up tomorrow. That'll cause a scene, I expect, but I will have to handle it. On the subject of psychology, I have done no revision for the past week. It just totally slipped my mind that I was supposed to be doing it! Even so, it seems like the grimoir is more important. I have decided to get on with that, and get into revision when it's finished. Things in this hospital are beginning to get more and more boring as they escalate. Just living day to day in an asylum is difficult, if you're sane!

9/4/99.

I missed psychology today. I will probably get into trouble for it, but I have had enough. Dr. Huff seems to think I "hear voices," and therefore I get treatment for symptoms that don't exist. As well as this, he is perpetually asking me about my sex life. There are things which I really want to keep secret, and at this rate, he is soon going to get on to Strangeways. I've discussed this before, but the situation is getting serious.

Ruth Kettle has set me up again. This time she sets it up deliberately to the public, that the police know that the Guerilla Press were responsible for riots and the bomb. I will now get set up for Broadmoor, even though I have been protesting my sanity for the past six years.

The good news, however, is that it has been established by Satanism that I wasn't actually responsible for torturing her, as she has claimed for the past twenty years. Even so, they are allowing her to use the T.V. to corrupt, and she is a seriously dodgy cunt. Vigilantes have said that she could be in trouble with them, as it was her who spread a false rumour that Desperadoes tortured her and fucked up the revolt against the Poll Tax. Still, what this fucker has been setting out to do is wind me up: aggro. She is quite likely to use the opportunity of being discredited in public in order to wind me up again. This is fair enough; well actually it isn't, but the staff are going to take it into their pathetic stupid and authoritarian little heads that Ruth Kettle is a figment of my imagination.

Anyway, now that she's been discredited, it means more support from guerrillas, and could mean another wave of revolution. This is obviously good news. Even if it doesn't, I have been persecuted a lot because of this false accusation, and I am owed a formal apology from a lot of people: for everything from conning Jenny into prostitution, to voodoo.

This is the end for Ruth Kettle now. How I did it, I don't know. Expecting post from my Dad tomorrow, and with Ruth Kettle losing her support from people like Class War, it could mean a wave of revolutionary consciousness through the C.C.A. propaganda group. I pick up my computer tomorrow, and I can get started on rewriting Volume 1. Despite having this idea, I still have to finish this booklet on Beelzebub. Things might be getting better.

11/4/99.

A very good day yesterday. Not as much mail as I had hoped for, though. A rejection letter from the Games publisher, saying that they liked the game but, due to their customers being aged between ten and fourteen, they would be unable to take copies. So I am going to have to try elsewhere. Something from the corrupt deposit office, and a catalogue for porn videos sent from Amsterdam. Both deserve some token description, so I will explain.

The letter from the copyright deposit office, A.T. Smail, is something that comes through the post every time I print a pamphlet. It basically just says that they've received the five copies that I sent them, and forwarded them to the main libraries. I was slightly disappointed that they apparently hadn't registered the R.P.R. system. It seems as if the Radical Presses Register isn't really taking off. I really think that I have had a lack of support due to the fact that I am disabled. I am considering writing them a letter.

About the catalogue of porn films: it was sent through an address that I found in a pornographic magazine. The advert was for "free sex lists," so I thought I'd write them a letter to see if there were any contacts. I've never seen a porn film, and I don't intend to start now, so I lent the thing to a friend on another Bungalow. I've also offered to lend him a tenner to buy one, but I don't know where that'll lead.

But the best letter I received yesterday was from 'Neoist Alliance', who are a situationist group based in London. They sent me some newsletters and stuff, with a note saying they liked the pamphlet. This is the first response from *Propaganda Groups*, and I am thinking about joining them in a full capacity; maybe in order to print pamphlets for them. I'll see how it goes.

Got the computer back yesterday. Apparently it only took an hour to fix, but there were a lot of things wrong with it. Now that it's back, I intend to complete the pamphlet on Beelzebub on the computer, and then get back on to Books 1 & 2 of Volume 1. I don't know how I coped without a computer for the past week, but I think I'll set it up tomorrow.

As well as all this going on, I bought a new toothbrush, some more toothpaste, some shampoo and a packet of condoms. I got myself some lettering at a very cheap price, which I will use to do the lettering in Volume 1, and also a new ink cartridge for the printer, a new T-shirt and a couple of books. One of the books was Rosemary's Baby, which I have wanted to read for a while, and the other was on Tutenkhamen, which will be useful for the game, if it ever gets set up and running.

I have asked my doctor about depression. Over the past few weeks I have been feeling very depressed. I am going to ask her for some mood-altering drugs. I just feel as if there is no way forward. I expected them to let me out a long time ago. I was originally sectioned eight years ago now, for putting a brick through a window. Since that I have never been medically discharged, even though I have been completely sane through most of my time of hospital. They just find excuses to keep me inside again, and again and again. All this is because the press insist on monitoring what I think. I believe that this makes me a political prisoner, set up by the State because of guerrilla activity to overthrow the Conservative Party State at the start of the decade. I now intend to escalate this crap from the press, by publicly organising the next event: "002 - The Millennium Bug." I know that this will stir the shit, but I have been under so much pressure to continue Strangeways that I think I should give them what they want.

Class War have become a faction of fascist sell outs, and they are never going to do anything to escalate revolution. The people are relying on me now. The revolution is an ongoing process and, if I can introduce the next generation to riot, as well as upholding my own generation, then I will be going something positive for change.

13/4/99.

The depletion of the environment is making itself apparent. There is rain, sleet and snow falling from the sky. It is a horrible day.

I sit here this rainy Tuesday listening to the radio. The T.V. is on the blink, and there is little to do, despite the psychological persecution that I will inevitably be put under as a result of listening to it. Received another rejection letter today, although I don't know who it was from. If I read the letter I sent, which has been returned, I might find out. Even so, it is depressing getting nothing but rejection letters. How long can this go on for? Anyway, having nothing left to write, I leave this for a month, on the day Nostradamus prophesied World War Three, to write a retrospective review of the year so far.

I now consider the idea of Stonehenge candles. It was the proposed means of raising funds in the pamphlet from the last Volume, *V. M. P.: a Statement ov Intent*. I am expecting a backdated D.L.A. cheque, and I thought that, instead of using money to print more pamphlets which are never going to sell, I could do better to commission a candlemaker to make, say 200 candles for me. These candles could be sold in a plastic zip bag, with a printed leaflet about Stonehenge and the significance of the candle itself.

These candles would be striped, with one stripe of purple designating a standing stone, and a stripe of black directly above it representing the space between each stone. This idea would be repeated to the height of the candle, representing the entire stone circle, starting and finishing at the Winter Solstice.

I feel that this project would be a better idea than spending more and more money trying to sell pamphlets, etc. This project will still involve some printing, as I will have to print a sheet to sell with the candle, about Stonehenge and the significance of the candle, and a leaflet to send to "alternative shops" to sell them.

200

At the same time, it occurs to me that I will have to find a list-broker for outlets. At present I am not sure how to do this, but with a little research it shouldn't be too difficult. But at the moment, I feel that selling them by mail order would be the best idea. For this reason, I will have to do an advert (something along the lines of the leaflet), and put it in some magazine like Green Anarchist.

Had an interesting day today. Printed a number of leaflets last night, to try to organise a shoplifting campaign to coincide with the millennium bug. It turned out that I had exactly enough A.A.A. leaflets to send to contacts, three leaflets more than I needed after sending out to all contacts, and three stamps left. I see all this, on April 13th, to be astrologically linked. It all seems like some sort of coincidence. Tonight I intend to forward a copy of 'e' to the Stonehenge campaign as a part of this run of coincidences. I might also write to the solicitors complaints address.

14/4/99.

Now that the games distribution people have decided not to take copies of 'e', there seems little point in printing it. I have got a book from the library today about 'running a business from home', so there may still be some point in printing it, and setting the Guerilla Press up as a business. I am currently thinking about setting up Cross Bootlegs Group in order to fund the Guerilla Press as a free distribution organisation. By this I mean printing literature to send out for free, and financing the idea through selling Dave Davey C.D.s. Assuming, of course, that he ever gets back in touch.

This idea inspires me. I am already sending out everything I print for free, and if I was to make a point about this, then I could build some sound practical support. The plan is this.

First I get the backdated D.L.A. cheque I have been waiting for. That should come in about two weeks. I use that to print, say, 200 C.D.s and a colour leaflet to try to sell them. I will probably do about 2,500 leaflets, This leaflet will specifically state that the C.D. is a benefit for the Guerilla Press. I will distribute these with a duplicate letter to the Free Information Network. If this C.D. sells, I can use the money to print more literature, including a leaflet saying it costs nothing to be put on our contacts list. Soon after that I should be looking at discharge, and should be free to organise benefit gigs. This will be going on simultaneously to the Radical Presses Register, which I will finance through my own pocket.

Additional funds may come from the book I finished today. It is a satire on the *Satanic Verses*, but still needs some editing. I have been reading through it tonight. I am actually very pleased with the book as it stands at the moment, although quite a lot of it has to be changed. Despite this, I am confident that I can get it published when it's edited. I really should make an effort to take revision more seriously, however. The exam is in two weeks.

That's about all that's happened today. Things move slowly in this place, but I have written to the solicitors complaints department, and I hope to be able to embark on a project to sue Ruth Kettle for breaching my copyright.

Refused my injection today on the grounds that I wanted to see my doctor beforehand. I look forward to another migraine when it eventually comes tomorrow.

TRUE STORIES FROM THE ARCHIVES OF SURVIVAL IN WEST YORKSHIRE

TERRY SIMPSON

B. had a dream that while a patient on a psyche ward, he'd died and his body was lying on a trolley in the hospital. A nurse came up with a clipboard, and apologetically explained that since he had not yet been discharged, he was not at liberty to die, and he would have to return until the proper paperwork was completed.

S. did not enamour himself to the professionals of Roundhay Wing, the psyche bit of St. James Hospital, when during one wild phase he donned a white jacket. Impersonating a doctor, he toured the wards doing impromptu ward rounds and discharging all the patients.

O. had been an outdoor pursuit instructor, and still had the climbing gear stashed in his second floor council flat. It seemed natural when he'd lost his keys in the flat one day, and locked himself in, to utilise this. It worked very well for him, but it did provoke a complaint to the council from the couple on the first floor, who were startled by the sight of a man suddenly abseiling past their living room window.

One day I was talking to D. at the centre when he produced an apple from his pocket and lit it up. A big plume of suspicious-smelling smoke arose. I looked on fascinated and he winked at me. "Chillum. Gives it a nice taste, and if we get busted I just eat the evidence."

G. was having one of his periodic highs, and was ushered into a little room to wait for the doctor to come and assess him. It was pretty bare, but there was a door inside the room with a sign on it that said "THIS DOOR MUST BE KEPT LOCKED AT ALL TIMES." And the first thing the doctor did on entering the room was to unlock it - crazy!

J. tells a story of taking acid in a house with friends, and going into a deep meditation. His friends thought it would be fun to pick him up and put him in the bedroom. He was so deeply gone he claims he had no idea what was happening. When he woke up he was in a room he'd never seen before, and alone. He freaked out completely, thinking he'd transmigrated back into the wrong body and become someone else.

M. drove her car on past the end of the road proper, onto the track, and finally the bare moor, swerving to avoid boulders, at one time following a rather startled rabbit. Reaching the top of Ilkley Moor, she tried to reverse the car, and abandoned it when she found she couldn't. She confessed what she'd done at a nursing home at the bottom of the hill, and a policeman gave her money which she spent in a nearby bar. The police were amazed at where the car had ended up, and it proved impossible to move under its own steam. They ended up air-lifting it off with a helicopter.

When A. was at Highroyds, a young woman on section was refused permission to attend her own wedding. She was furious, and complaining bitterly in the smoke room about this. An older woman took a more philosophical view. "Don't worry about it, love. I wish someone had stopped me getting to my wedding..."

A. (to psychiatric nurse): Are you mad too?

Nurse : I think I'm just dreaming I'm a psychiatric nurse, and that one day someone will give me an injection, and I'll wake up and realise this has all just been a bad dream.

These stories are all true, or so they told me.

CUCKOOS DON'T MAKE NESTS
NICK BLINKO

Curious? I'm furious!/ Fly Pie/ The Bladder ladder/ Crazy baby/ Dr. Fay Talatie/ flaying with Pyre/ Sphere Shaped room/ A stipulative character/ Dolls of IDOLS/ 1000000%/ Threaded Headed thread headed/ Dr. Tiny Stipend/ Ice- olated/ Mr. Wreck Tangle/ empty bone in the brain/ boney brain/ passionate Assassins. Associates/ Secret scarlet stolen ego/ meagre ogre/ see the wretch retch/ A miracle; America!/ the Mental Health Act Commissioners control patients by pulling levers and the awesome but awful descendants of levers/ I did we stint as a Saint once/ where they don't say where/ punlocked/ mediocre medicine/ I can smell her thinking/ Eelectricity/ Skeleton of a thought/ Passionate Patient/ the feeded seas/ Clouds resembling e.g. giant birds, become huge versions of what they looked like/ imbibe bile, umbilical bile BiBlical bile/ Ironic moronic/ I don't want to DIE anymore/ quietly clapping/ after breaking a bone in her ego/ Pactor/ Just before I died/ the doors of the domes/ Scared for life/ muffled thud baffled thunder/ A gramme of germs (10 grammes of germs)/ Antique Inquisition/ Corner-cutting coroner/ wretched, squalid/ In the charnel's channels/ deeply gloomy/ Photo Pathos/ garbled marble message/ mad in the head - mad in the heart/ They put me in a grey cell/ the cigarettes blue hue/ Insanitorium/ in order to ignite his cognition.

Union being/ murmuring mermaids/ chime machine/ immeasurably miserable/ virtual suicide/ Sinmaster/ golden giddy/ Vowing to be vomiting on such and such a date/ the orphan donor/ muttering nutter/ violent ties - violent eyes/ babybody/ curious in the cradle/ the embodiment of disembodiment/ the findings of the foundlings/ The White Plague/ illdefined state of mind/ muddied mind/ dragon flying diagonally/ the hunted haunted/ my eyes are spies/ nil by word of mouth/ that's not collusion that's a collision/ the role would ripen/ soldier spiders/ Rumblebrain/ Mister Monster/ Zoozones/ Plush Fish/ Side by Suicide/ Mr. Sister/ she hanged her husband/ vomit Pride Pie/ Earlier Aeons/ Geologician-glacierologist/ crotchety in the corner/ such dreamy dramas Dr./ Unscathed satyrs/ Unscathed Martyrs/ accused of maliciously wounding his life/ Dr. Frictionfractionfunction/ crimminalanimmal/ amazing wonderment & astonishing awesome joyousness/ craggy and maggoty/ Argue Target/ Pity guilty/ maroon moron/ Dr. Ceoliacanth, expert in living fossils/ Paean to Pain/ Ear Sea/ Callous Palace/ the crux of the crucible (Crucifix)/ sought after laughter/ future funeral/ the monitoring conspiracy/ groan town/ A consignment of puzzlement/ puzzling pizzles/ there was no opposition to the vile opposition/ The Ladies' ideas.

Bemuseum/ Shivering silver slivers/ Brawn & Bread/ Egg-Cracker/ gush & gape/ Dream Disease/ the heart which boasts blasphemy/ Admiral Abominable/ & then the exonerated exited.

Amnometre - for measuring animosity/ Nervevalve - for detecting ferocity/ salvotalie - for listening to love/ thought Order - distractor/ Augmented fianchetto detector/ Nocturnally extracted - madness/ Divert tears to - lunar re-alignment/ gross moral torpitude - festering in a globule/ the 99th sense - uncompartalizable in anyway/ the horrification - unlimnable/ 9 Million murders ago - you can't suppress it/ inkpen of iniquity - dispersed/ manipulate - cynical contrivances.

Murder monster murder a monster.

HEAVEN IS A MAD PLACE ON EARTH
SIMON MORRIS

The 'Mad Pride' virus is now loose and the term will no doubt begin to enter common currency over the next few years, leading to its eventual recuperation.

Mad Pride is the first 'survivor movement' that's really appealed to me. Mental health resource users are now actively encouraged by statutory health authorities and by many charities to get involved in improving the psychiatric system - firstly purely as volunteers, and now increasingly in paid employment. This is all well and good, but it defines us forever as the (ex) 'patient' - it defines us only in terms of our involvement with the control system that is institutional psychiatry. A far greater and much more pleasant part of our lives is made up of drinking, shagging, drugging it, takeaway curries, blagging vast amounts of loony benefit, and myriad forms of (hopefully completely out there) creativity. For me, Mad Pride takes the user movement into a higher realm of political awareness and the challenging of social roles.

Anyone who's ever read anything about shamanism will recognise certain parallels with what's termed 'mental illness' in modern western culture. The model of the shaman in our society is often claimed to be rock stars (Jim Morrison springs to mind - unfortunately). Mad Pride offers the slogan 'Madness is the new rock 'n' roll!' There really is so much that's positive and exciting about 'illnesses' like 'schizophrenia'. All of us who've experienced 'deep sea fishing' will know the sensation of heightened awareness, of consciousness enhanced far better than LSD could ever do it, of feelings of wonder and terror that can't be verbalised... and then have these visions which effortlessly outstrip the alienation of daily life dismissed as 'delusion' by some fucking shrink. Nearly everything that's 'bad' about madness is caused by the reactions of the restrained, shrivelled and grey majority to someone near them being beautifully crazy and alive!

I was always a mad kid. At junior school I had a punk band called The Headbangers - my stage name was 'Mental Moz' and I tried to live up to it. We did a gig in our back garden and threw buckets of water around like on Tiswas.

I was always mad because I never wanted to be part of the shitty straight world - what kind of pervert actually wants to go out to some job they hate day after day, kneel to a boss they hate, buy the right car/ right clothes/ right computer/ right CDs and still feel empty? Fuck that con!

I was always mad - bunking off early from school when I was 15 to go home and stare at a self-constructed dream machine while tripping out to Throbbing Gristle and Butthole Surfers records. And spending the 15 years since then making demented, wilfully unlistenable records of my own.

I was always mad, and it was a lovely thrill to realise that there were plenty of mad girls out there who liked mad boys and mad sex. I still love them all - even the *really* crazy ones.

I was always mad, and OK, being caught by the psychiatric system was no fun and sometimes the enhanced awareness that comes when I'm VERY mad can be a bit much to cope with. But I'm still glad to be mad - beautiful, clinching evidence of concrete outsiderdom (my tattoo reads 'ONE PER CENT'). Well-meaning halfwits who spout on about 'social inclusion' are barking up the wrong tree as far as I'm concerned. One campaign I would support would be a Mad Pride Campaign to Repeal the British Licensing Laws Immediately. So many of us are insomniacs and it'd be great to be able to go down the pub and meet all your nutty mates at 4 am. The hours are a clear-cut case of discrimination against the psychiatrically challenged at present!

The user movement is currently being empowered to learn to hold meetings and enter the more than 36 chambers of bureaucracy. Mad Pride empowers us to rave in space at the very least, and at best to take our dreams for reality. This train is bound for the Western Lands - hold on tight.

I was always mad - I hope I always will be. My crazy life is wonderful. The 'sane' really don't know what they're missing.

ABOUT THE AUTHORS

FRANK BANGAY was born in Wandsworth, South London in 1951. He left school at 15, and went to evening classes a few years later to brush up on his grammar. He started writing poetry in 1972. A co-founder of Survivors Poetry, he is currently involved with a survivor writing group at Core Arts in Hackney. He continues to write and perform, and aims to keep doing so despite dodgy spelling.

NICK BLINKO was born in 1961. Since 1980 he has been singer, guitarist and songwriter in the acclaimed punk trio Rudimentary Peni, whose records include *Death Church*, *Cacophony* and *Pope Adrian 37th Psychristiatric*. His paintings have been exhibited all over the world, and his first novel, *The Primal Screamer*, was published in 1995.

LUTHER BLISSETT is a man or woman of multiple origins. S/he allegedly invented three-sided football, which dissolves the homoerotic/homophobic bipolarity of the two-sided game, thus breaking down the very basis of capitalist organisation.

STEPHEN BUDD was born in Somerset in 1965, educated at Wells Cathedral School, Somerset, graduated from Bristol Polytechnic in 1988 as a property surveyor and is married with three children. He was diagnosed with bi-polar affective disorder in spring of 1999 and subsequently sectioned to hospital on a number of occasions over the next six months. When he discovered that manic depression tended to affect articulate, intelligent and creative people, he wrote his piece in this book.

LOUISE C. was born in London in 1963. In the early 80s she lived with the Kill Your Pet Puppy anarcho fanzine collective. She was in various bands including the obscure Mental Disorder and Hysteria Ward. She loves the Levellers, her pet budgie and her daughter, Rebecca.

TERRY CONWAY was quarried in Islington in 1952. For the last sixteen years he has lived in Hackney with his wife and two children. In 1994 he became co-founder and chair for three years of Hackney Patients Council. The naive fool now likes to believe that he is challenging the system from within as a social worker.

TED CURTIS was born close to the north-eastern boundary of Ethnic Somerset in the heady days of 1983, when other stuff was making the news. A fish-designer by trade, he is covered in tattoos and scars like many trendies. Following recent events, he is now with the angels and the baby Jesus.

ROBERT DELLAR, born in Watford in 1964, is 5'10" and rides a pushbike. Since 1987 he has worked for various Mind affiliations, most recently in Southwark. He is editor of the punk short story collection *Gobbing, Pogoing and Gratuitous Bad Language* and co-author of the novel *Seaton Point*.

FATMA DURMUSH was born in 1959. She has spent most of her life trying to write. In doing this she did not get her degree. She has been published in The Big Issue over 100 times. She has been on the radio, and also in She and Daily Express. Her prolific writing includes poetry, plays and short stories.

MICHAEL HOWLETT was born in 1963 in Huddersfield. He regrets being lumbered with the same name as a well-known campaigner against psychiatric patients' rights, a co-incidence which encourages his mates to take the piss out of him.

ESTHER LESLIE is a Walter Benjamin scholar with a post at Birkbeck College. Her forthcoming publications include *Walter Benjamin: Overpowering Conformism* (Pluto) and *Hollywood Flatlands: Critical Theory, the Avantgarde & Animation* (Verso). She is on the editorial boards of the journals *Revolutionary History* and *Historical Materialism*.

JAMES MACDOUGALL was born in Andover, Hampshire in 1968. He learnt through years of experience, chance meetings and of course the odd aspirin or two that the mentally ill, disabled, and even Helen Keller prove through perseverance that the paranoid can achieve what the social norm cannot. Daydream nation we love you, and all the twisted things you make us do.

DEBBIE MCNAMARA was born playing air chords on the banjo, delivered by her auntie in Manchester. A lifetime of discovering her purpose quickly ensued, including teaching at posh colleges in Harrogate, being the pivot worker for early Survivors' Poetry and selling beer as a full-time occupation in Birmingham. She now works for the Patients' Council in a hospital where she was once a patient, organises gigs and studies pastry-making.

THE MENTAL PATIENTS UNION formed after a 'user' action at Paddington Day Hospital in 1972 and was based in North Kensington.

A few years later a branch was set up in Hackney. (Frank Bangay adds: "I first met Eric Irwin in 1980 when I first became involved with the survivor movement. Eric was born in Belfast in the early 1920s. He was a survivor with many years' experience in psychiatric institutions, and a tireless campaigner and activist, until he died in 1987. He was well-read, extremely knowledgeable and had a wonderful sense of humour. He was once sick over R.D. Laing at a party; the pair are now having a debate up in heaven.")

SIMON MORRIS is the lead shapeshifter for mad Blackpool punk band Ceramic Hobs, whose records include *Psychiatric Underground* and *Straight Outta Rampton*. On November 25, 1970, at the peak of his brilliant literary career, he astonished the world by committing ritual suicide, or hara-kiri, by disembowelment.

HUGH MULHALL, conceived in Liverpool, was born in London on 23rd November 1963 to Irish parents. He studied at Liverpool and Thames Polytechnics, and has on two occasions been admitted to psychiatric hospital.

EDWARD MURRAY was born in Donegal, Ireland in 1959. He trained as a metalworker/welder before moving to London in 1983 to work in that trade. After a family tragedy he returned to education and graduated in Law from the London School of Economics in 1993. He is currently working as a volunteer mental health advocate at the Maudsley Hospital, Southwark.

HANNE OLSEN was born in Elsinore, Denmark, in 1964. At 24 she came to Lancaster, at 26 went to live in Glasgow and at 28 in London. As well as writing stories she is part of Kingston User Forum (0181 547 2319).

CHRIS P. found his mental breakdown a particularly creative period after the band he was in, Silverfish, split up. He joined the bands Headbutt and Copyright. He has also been published in the Spare Change anthology *Gobbing, Pogoing and Gratuitous Bad Language*. He is now settling down to the relative sanity of fatherhood.

MARK ROBERTS is a survivor activist and a committed loony who has been working in mental health for the last ten years. Before that he was a rhythm guitarist in a soul band and also did some low-level freelance journalism. He still manages to write the odd song. Now he works on campaigns run by disabled people and mental health survivors. Currently the main issue we are working on is fighting the fascist new Mental Health Act which seeks to force often harmful drugs on people. Mark is a member of the UK-based company Mad Pride.

PETE SHAUGHNESSY, born in Saff London in 1962, started Reclaim Bedlam in 1997 after a dream of inspiration at his Mum's. He says: "I have to be as I am, and if that is deemed Madness, then so be it and I'll be damned." Reclaim Bedlam has organised five Direct Actions against hypocrisy and/or state coercion. More are planned.

TERRY SIMPSON lives in Leeds with a piano. He works for the UK Advocacy Network, and his heroes/heroines include Carol Batton and Robin Hood. His ambitions are to write the definitive survivor novel, free the world from mental health oppression, and still have plenty of time to sing.

TIM TELSA is the archetypal psychiatric patient. He suffers from delusions of state persecution and big brother. When he is not causing a management problem by refusing medication, he runs a highly disturbing self-publishing group. On one occasion, when he tried to set up a cult, the police were called in by a local bookseller, and all copies of his publication on Mars rockets were confiscated by the hospital. Write to him c/o The Guerilla Press: B.M. Betelguise, London WC1N 3XX.

BEN WATSON is a music critic. His books include *Frank Zappa: The Negative Dialectics of Poodle Play* (1994) and *Derek Bailey & the Story of Free Improvisation* (forthcoming). His Mad Pride essay is a second attempt to understand the deplorable glory of madness; the first appeared in his *Art, Class & Cleavage: Quantulumcunque Concerning Materialist Esthetix* (1998).

MAD AND UNREASONABLE INDEX

217

221

Printed in the United Kingdom
by Lightning Source UK Ltd.
113823UKS00001B/132